Ethical Issues
in Preventive Medicine

NATO ASI Series
Advanced Science Institutes Series

A Series presenting the results of activities sponsored by the NATO Science Committee, which aims at the dissemination of advanced scientific and technological knowledge, with a view to strengthening links between scientific communities.

The Series is published by an international board of publishers in conjunction with the NATO Scientific Affairs Division

A	Life Sciences	Plenum Publishing Corporation
B	Physics	London and New York
C	Mathematical and Physical Sciences	D. Reidel Publishing Company Dordrecht and Boston
D	Behavioural and Social Sciences	Martinus Nijhoff Publishers Dordrecht/Boston/Lancaster
E	Applied Sciences	
F	Computer and Systems Sciences	Springer-Verlag Berlin/Heidelberg/New York
G	Ecological Sciences	

Series D: Behavioural and Social Sciences – No. 26

Ethical Issues in Preventive Medicine

Editor:
Spyros Doxiadis, MD
President
Foundation for Research in Childhood
42, Amalias Street
Athens 105 58, Greece

Editorial Committee:

Roger Blaney, MD
Senior Lecturer, Dept. of Community Medicine,
Queen's University, Belfast, Northern Ireland, UK

Lucien Karhausen, MD
Officer of the Commission of the EEC, Brussels, Belgium

Heleen Terborgh-Dupuis, PhD.
Professor of Ethics, Faculty of Medicine
Leiden University, Leiden, The Netherlands

Susie Stewart
Technical Editor, Glasgow, Scotland, UK

1985 **Martinus Nijhoff Publishers**
Dordrecht / Boston / Lancaster
Published in cooperation with NATO Scientific Affairs Division

Proceedings of the NATO Advanced Research Workshop on Ethical Issues in Preventive Medicine, Athens, Greece, January 10-12, 1985, organized by:
The NATO Science Council and **The Foundation for Research in Childhood,**
in collaboration with **The Commission of the European Economic Communities**
and **The Panel of Social Medicine and Epidemiology of the EEC**

Library of Congress Cataloging in Publication Data

NATO Advanced Research Workshop on Ethical Issues
  in Preventive Medicine (1985 : Athens, Greece)
  Ethical issues in preventive medicine.

  (NATO ASI series. Series D, Behavioural and social
sciences ; no. 26)
  "Proceedings of the NATO Advanced Research Workshop
on Ethical Issues in Preventive Medicine, Athens,
Greece, January 10-12, 1985"--T.p. verso.
  Organized by the NATO Science Council and other
agencies.
  "Published in cooperation with NATO Scientific Affairs
Division."
  Includes index.
  1. Medical ethics--Congresses. 2. Medicine, Preventive
--Congresses. I. Doxiadés, Spyros. II. NATO Science
Council. III. North Atlantic Treaty Organization.
Scientific Affairs Division. IV. Title. V. Series.
  [DNLM: 1. Ethics, Medical--congresses. 2. Preventive
Medicine--congresses. WA 108 N279e 1985]
  R725.5.N38 1985   174'.2   85-18913
  ISBN 90-247-3232-8

ISBN 90-247-3232-8 (this volume)
ISBN 90-247-2688-3 (series)

Distributors for the United States and Canada: Kluwer Boston, Inc., 190 Old Derby Street, Hingham, MA 02043, USA

Distributors for the UK and Ireland: Kluwer Academic Publishers, MTP Press Ltd, Falcon House, Queen Square, Lancaster LA1 1RN, UK

Distributors for all other countries: Kluwer Academic Publishers Group, Distribution Center, P.O. Box 322, 3300 AH Dordrecht, The Netherlands

All rights reserved. No part of this publication may be reproduced, stored in a retrieval system, or transmitted, in any form or by any means, mechanical, photocopying, recording, or otherwise, without the prior written permission of the publishers,
Martinus Nijhoff Publishers, P.O. Box 163, 3300 AD Dordrecht, The Netherlands

Copyright © 1985 by Martinus Nijhoff Publishers, Dordrecht

Printed in The Netherlands

PREFACE

The first suggestions and exchange of ideas for this Workshop began about two years ago when, at the invitation of Professor E Bennett, Director of Health and Safety of the Commission of the European Communities and Professor W W Holland of the Panel of Social Medicine and Epidemiology of the EEC, I asked the Panel to sponsor a project for the study of Ethical Issues in Preventive Medicine. The Panel gave its approval and support and asked Dr L Karhausen, Dr R Blaney, and me to undertake the planning. Since then we have had several meetings in Brussels and have added Professor Heleen Terborgh-Dupuis and Mrs Susie Stewart to our small planning team.

The Planning Committee invited many experts to collaborate with us on the project and, as can be seen from the list of participants, they represent many scientific disciplines and many countries. About a year ago we also asked for the help and sponsorship of the NATO Science Council which was generously given. The culmination of our efforts was the Workshop held in Athens in January 1985, the proceedings of which are contained in the present book.

The members of the Planning Committee and the participants at the Workshop would like to express thanks to Mr H Durand, Secretary General for NATO Scientific Affairs and Dr M di Lullo, Programme Director of NATO Scientific Affairs and to Professor Bennett and Professor Holland for all the moral and financial support they have given to this project.

Spyros Doxiadis
Athens
June 1985

CONTENTS

	Page
Preface	v
List of participants	ix

Session I
Chairman: Dr A Campbell — 1

1 Introductory talk — 1
Dr S Doxiadis

2 Medical ethics and moral philosophy — 5
Dr L Karhausen

Session II — 11
Chairman: Professor D Trihopoulos

3 Evolution and mutation in medical ethics — 11
Professor G R Dunstan

4 Theoretical basis of disease prevention — 19
Dr R Blaney

Session III — 24
Chairman: Professor D Beauchamp

5 Development of preventive medicine and health promotion — 25
Dr A H M Kerkhoff

6 Ethical aspects of public health legislation and the role of the state — 32
Dr G Pinet

Subsidiary presentation — 36
Oregon health decisions
Dr R Crawshaw

Session IV — 42
Chairman: Professor O Harlem

7 Ethical aspects of the economics of prevention — 42
Dr M Bungener

8 Ethical issues in descriptive and analytical epidemiology and in primary prevention — 46
Professor E G Knox

Session V — 54
Chairman: Dr D Roy

9 Ethical issues in trials of prevention — 54
Dr T Strasser

10 Ethical issues of health promotion, health education, and behavioural control 59
Professor L Eisenberg

Session VI 61
Chairman: Professor S Gorovitz

11 Ethical issues in the activities of mass media communication in health education 65
Claire Rayner

12 Ethical issues in occupational health 72
Sir Edward Pochin

Subsidiary presentation 74
Role of the company physician
Professor Rainer Muller

Session VII 78
Chairman: Dr R Nicholson

13 Ethics, prevention, and child health 78
Professor E A Sand

14 Ethical issues in mass screening procedures 84
Professor P Riis

Session VIII 90
Chairman: Professor R Veatch

15 Ethical aspects of population control 90
Professor H Terborgh-Dupuis

16 Methods and procedures of ethical control 95
Dr J F Martin

Closing remarks 102

Index 104

LIST OF PARTICIPANTS

Professor Dan E Beauchamp
Department of Public Policy and
Administration
School of Public Health
The University of North Carolina at
Chapel Hill
263 Rosenau Building, 201 Chapel Hill
North Carolina 27514-6201, USA

Dr Roger Blaney
Institute of Clinical Science
The Queen's University of Belfast
Grosvenor Road
Belfast BT12 6BJ
Northern Ireland

Dr Martine Bungener
Economist
LEGOS
Universite de Paris 1X Dauphine
Place du Mal de Lattre de Tassigny
75016 Paris
France

Reverend Dr Alastair Campbell
Department of Christian Ethics and
Practical Theology
University of Edinburgh
New College
The Mound
Edinburgh EH1 2LX
Scotland

Professor Cipriano Canosa
Ciudad Sanitaria de la Seguridad Social
"La Fe"
Instituto Nacional de la Salud
Avenida Campanar 21
Valencia 9
Spain

Mrs Pelaghia Cottaridi
Sociologist
Foundation for Research in Childhood
42 Amalias Street
Athens 105 58
Greece

Dr Ralph Crawshaw
Psychiatrist
2525 N W Lovejoy Street
Suite 404
Portland
Oregon 97210, USA

Ms Panayiota Dalas-Voria
Doctor-at-Law
Department of Hygiene and
Epidemiology
University of Athens Medical School
Athens 115 27
Greece

Mr Nicos Dimou
Writer
15-17 Tsoha Street
Athens 115 21
Greece

Professor Spyros Doxiadis
Paediatrician
President
Foundation for Research in Childhood
42 Amalias Street
Athens 105 58
Greece

Professor G R Dunstan
Department of Theology, University of
Exeter
Queen's Building
The University
Exeter EX4 4QH
England

Professor Leon Eisenberg
Department of Social Medicine and
Health Policy
Harvard Medical School
25 Shattuck Street
Boston
Massachussetts 02115, USA

Professor Samuel Gorovitz
Department of Philosophy
Division of Arts and Humanities
University of Maryland
College Park 20742
Maryland, USA

Professor O K Harlem
Paediatrician
Editor, The Journal of the Norwegian
Medical Association
Inkognitogt 26
Oslo 2
Norway

Professor Olivier Jeanneret
Institute of Social and Preventive
Medicine
University of Geneva
27 Quai Charles-Page
CH-1211 Geneva 4
Switzerland

Dr Lucien Karhausen
Commission of the European
Communities
Directorate of Health and Safety
Batiment Jean Monnet
Plateau du Kirchberg
L-2920 Luxembourg

Dr A H M Kerkhoff
Director
Public Health Services
Warmonderweg 3
2334 AA Leiden
The Netherlands

Professor E G Knox
Health Services Research Centre
Department of Social Medicine
The Medical School
Edgbaston
Birmingham B15 2TJ
England

Professor Ioanna Lambiri-Dimaki
Sociologist
School of Law
University of Athens
20 Kanari Street
Athens 106 74
Greece

Dr Dimitra Makrynioti
Sociologist
Foundation for Research in Childhood
42 Amalias Street
Athens 105 58
Greece

Dr Jean Martin
Institute of Social and Preventive
Medicine
University of Lausanne
CH-1011 Lausanne
Switzerland

Professor Rainer Müller
Physician, Sociologist
University of Bremen
Bibliothekstrasse
Postfach 330440
Bremen
West Germany

Professor Yunus Mumuftu
Paediatrician
Hacettepe University
Ankara
Turkey

Dr Sheena Nakou
Paediatrician
Institute of Child Health
Athens 115 27
Greece

Dr Richard Nicholson
Institute of Medical Ethics
Tavistock House North
Tavistock Square
London WC1H 9LG
England

Dr Genevieve Pinet
Regional Officer for Health Legislation
World Health Organisation
8 Scherfigsvej
DK-2100 Copenhagen
Denmark

Sir Edward Pochin
Physician
National Radiological Protection Board
Chilton, Didcot
Oxfordshire OX11 ORQ
England

Mrs Claire Rayner
Nurse, Journalist
Holly Wood House
Roxborough Avenue
Harrow-on-the-Hill
Middlesex HO1 3BU
England

Professor Povl Riis
Medical-Gastroenterological Department
Herlev University Hospital
DK-2730 Herlev
Denmark

Professor David Roy
Center of Bioethics
Clinical Research Institute of Montreal
110 Avenue des Pins Quest
Montreal
Quebec H2W 1R7
Canada

Professor Alfred Sand
Universite Libre de Bruxelles
Campus Erasme
School of Public Health
Route de Lennik
B-1070 Brussels
Belgium

Mrs Susie Stewart
Technical Editor
34 Rowan Road
Dumbreck
Glasgow G41 5BZ
Scotland

Dr T Strasser
Department of Social and Preventive Medicine
University of Geneva
27 Quai Charles-Page
CH-1211 Geneva 4
Switzerland

Mr Nicolas Tatsis
Sociologist
Department of Political Science
University of Athens
19 Omirou Street
Athens 106 72
Greece

Professor Heleen Terborgh-Dupuis
METAMEDICA
Faculty of Medicine
p/a Pathologisch Laboratorium
Rijksuniversiteit Leiden
Postbus 9603
2300 RC Leiden
The Netherlands

Professor Gianni Tognoni
Laboratory of Clinical Pharmacology
Instituto di Ricerche Farmacologiche
"Mario Negri"
Via Eritrea 62
20157 Milan
Italy

Professor Dimitris Trihopoulos
Department of Hygiene and Epidemiology
School of Medicine
Athens University
Athens 115 27
Greece

Dr Helen Valassi-Adam
Paediatrician
Athens University Paediatric Clinic
Aghia Sophia Children's Hospital
Athens 115 27
Greece

Professor Robert Veatch
Joseph and Rose Kennedy Institute of Ethics
Georgetown University
Washington DC 20057, USA

Dr Lambrini Veloyianni-Moutsopoulou
Attorney-at-Law and Bioethicist
38 Bizaniou Street
Ioannina
Greece

Dr Meropi Violaki
Honorary Director General
Ministry of Health
2 Dimaki Street
Athens
Greece

The Very Reverend Archmandrite Dr A Zakopoulos
Dean, Archdiocese of Athens
Professor, Institute of Education
Patras 36, Sozopoleos Street
Athens 104 46
Greece

Dr Luke Zander
Senior Lecturer
General Practice Teaching Unit
St Thomas's Hospital Medical School
80 Kennington Road
London SE11 4TH
England

INTRODUCTORY TALK

SPYROS DOXIADIS

FOUNDATION FOR RESEARCH IN CHILDHOOD, ATHENS

Good morning and welcome again. It is a great pleasure to have you here and thank you for coming. I would now like to introduce the Chairman of the first session of the workshop. The Reverend Dr Alastair Campbell is Senior Lecturer in the Department of Christian Ethics and Practical Theology in the University of Edinburgh. He is a teacher, researcher, Minister of the Church of Scotland, author of several books and articles on medical ethics and a former editor of the Journal of Medical Ethics.

DR CAMPBELL (CHAIRMAN)

Thank you. I thought it was very good of the organisers of the symposium to decide to have a non-English speaker as the first chairman! Apparently those of us in Scotland do speak English rather more clearly than some others south of the border, and there is one thing that I would like to say at the beginning, in view of the fact that the conference language is English. I hope that people will not hesitate to say if they have difficulty in understanding those of us who have the advantage of having the mother tongue, if not the motherland, as English, and will insist that we speak clearly to improve communication between us all. We have a great privilege as English speakers in not having to worry about language, even although we do have some problems with our fellow English speakers at times. I will now ask Dr Doxiadis to give his introductory talk.

DR DOXIADIS

I would like to begin by explaining why we started this venture. There are three personal reasons for my interest in the subject of our work which will explain why I took the initiative to gather you here today.

The first reason is that about 20 years ago the Institute of Child Health of which at the time I was President, received a grant from the US National Institutes of Health to support our research into neonatal jaundice, and one of the conditions of the grant was that our Institute should establish an Ethical Review Committee to examine this and other research projects and proposals. Since then, ethical issues in research involving human subjects have become one of my main interests.

Secondly, since I have been a paediatrican for 40 years, it is natural, or perhaps inevitable, that I should become concerned with health promotion and disease prevention equally or even more than with treatment of illness. This has focussed my attention on problems arising out of these kinds of medical activities.

The third reason for my concern was that I became, some years ago, Minister of Health in Greece and I was for four years responsible for planning the health services of this country. This increased my awareness of the responsibilities of Government in planning and implementing programmes which raised many questions of an ethical nature.

When my term as Minister came to an end, I had more time for reading and thinking on the ethical issues involved in health promotion and disease prevention. I could not, however, find a whole book or even an extensive review devoted to this particular topic. Among the few articles some of the best were written by members of our workshop here. Furthermore, since almost all the writings were the work of ethicists, philosophers, and theologians, the point of view of medical people, concerned with public health, with planning, and with clinical practice was not clearly presented.

I started then to ask myself if an exchange of views and a book on ethical issues in preventive medicine could justify the expenditure of time and money it would entail. In the last 20 years, whole books, special journals, and congresses have been devoted to ethics in medical practice. It is not particularly strange or unexpected that writers, medical or otherwise, have been more interested in ethical problems arising out of treatment, of the one-to-one doctor to patient relationship that is the norm in medical practice. Doctors, patients, and the public in general have always preferred short-term satisfaction and short-term results to long-term social benefits. Thus I came to the conclusion that ethical issues in health promotion, health care, and disease prevention did deserve special attention because they were so different and equally or more important than similar issues in therapeutic medicine.

Moral problems in therapeutic medicine differ in various ways from those in health promotion and preventive medicine, and this second group is, in my view, more important since ignorance or indifference in this field of thought may have more serious consequences, more long-term results, and may affect many more people. Let me outline six of the important differences between therapeutic and preventive medicine from an ethical point of view.

First, in therapeutic medicine, one person or small numbers of people present the health problem. In preventive medicine, much larger numbers are involved. If an unethical decision is taken, therefore, it will affect many more people.

Secondly, in therapeutic medicine, the person or persons are ill when they present the problem. In preventive medicine, the subjects are usually healthy or apparently healthy. If an unethical decision is taken, therefore, it will affect people who have been previously entirely or apparently healthy, not ill.

Thirdly, the responsibility in therapeutic medicine is usually vested in one doctor or a small number of doctors or other health professionals. In this context, the responsibility of the state for ethical matters is very remote, if it exists at all. In preventive medicine, on the other hand, the responsibility of the state is often considerable. The community physician or health planner is rarely in direct contact with the subjects of his work and may, therefore, feel less responsible for his decisions. The problems of abortion, of euthanasia, of the mentally defective newborn presented in a clinical situation with an individual patient will appear very different from consideration of similar problems in a large anonymous population.

Fourthly, in therapeutic medicine the results of a decision are usually assessed within a few days, weeks, or months of a consultation. The results of decisions in preventive medicine frequently take a much longer time to evaluate. Again the responsibility is remote, and it may, therefore, tend to be forgotten.

Fifthly, in therapeutic medicine the criteria of success or failure are easily defined – death or life, an additional life or not, interruption of pregnancy or not, transplantation or not. In preventive medicine, the criteria of success or failure are defined much less easily or clearly because there are so many factors involved. Here again, this complexity of aetiological or contributing factors may tend to lessen the feeling of responsibility in those making the decisions.

Lastly, while decisions in therapeutic medicine are usually independent of the cultural, social, and economic background of the subject, many decisions in preventive medicine affect disadvantaged groups with inadequate knowledge of their own rights and of the consequences of possible courses of action. Our responsibility to protect the rights of such groups is great.

This then is the background to my feelings that a workshop entirely devoted to ethical issues in preventive medicine would be worthwhile. The workshop, rather than congress, format gives us freedom, during our discussions and later, to change even the title we have chosen – we may decide, for example, that it is more appropriate to describe the subject as ethical issues in health care, health promotion, or health policy.

To try to set up this workshop, I approached first, through the kind offices of Professor Trihopoulos, the Commission of the European Communities, and I presented my views to the Panel of Social Medicine and Epidemiology. They accepted the suggestion that they should sponsor the undertaking and they asked Dr Lucien Karhausen and Dr Roger Blaney to work with me in planning the workshop and subsequent publications. We then invited Dr Heleen Terborgh-Dupuis to join the Planning Committee and Mrs Susie Stewart to act as Technical Editor. The five of us have worked together, meeting on several occasions in Brussels, and we have chosen the main speakers and participants here today.

At one point there were some budgetary difficulties in the Commission and this compelled us to approach the Science Council of NATO for funding, again through the kind offices of Professor Trihopoulos. The response was favourable, and thanks to their contribution and that of the Foundation for Research in Childhood, based in Athens, we have been able to meet the expenses of the workshop.

There is a good representation of countries within the 10 countries of the European Community and of the 14 countries in NATO. Two or three countries are not included because we were unable to find a representative interested in this rather new field of ethical issues in preventive medicine. The representation of disciplines is not so balanced. There is a majority of medical doctors but this may be appropriate since doctors are often less sensitive to this particular topic and are perhaps more able to influence decisions on health matters taken by governments or other agencies. Represented here also are the separate disciplines of philosophy, ethics, theology, sociology, public health, economics, law, and journalism.

We decided to confine our discussions to ethical issues in preventive medicine in the developed countries of which those present here have direct personal experience. The problems and practice of prevention in the developing countries are of great importance but they are very different, and we felt that if we tried to deal also with these, it would be rather presumptuous. It would also have meant a much larger number of participants and too broad a scope of subject to cover effectively in the workshop.

Our aim in this whole undertaking is to make everyone concerned with health promotion and disease prevention and with planning and implementing health care policies – be they doctors, other health professionals, leaders of public opinion, members of parliaments and governments, employees of health ministries, journalists – more aware of and more sensitive to ethical issues and ethical problems in preventive medicine. I hope we will have a very productive meeting.

ADDITIONAL INTRODUCTORY COMMENTS

DR CAMPBELL

Before we begin with the first formal paper of the meeting, we will hear a general word from Dr Karhausen on behalf of the Commission of the European Communities and from Dr Pinet on behalf of the World Health Organisation.

DR KARHAUSEN

I would just like to add a few words to what Dr Doxiadis has said. The meeting we are holding here is part of a response to a request from the European Parliament to the Commission to undertake some work in the field of medical ethics and patients' rights. The first project in this area was carried out by Professor Knox whose report on confidentiality in medicine has recently been published. This workshop and the subsequent publications forms the second stage of the response to the European Parliament's request. On behalf of the Commission, I would like to record our thanks to Dr Doxiadis and the Foundation for Research in Childhood for organising the meeting. Dr Doxiadis has done most of the preparatory work and without him we would not all be here today.

DR PINET

I am grateful for the opportunity to say a few words on behalf of the Regional Office for Europe of the World Health Organisation and in particular our Regional Director, Dr Azban. We would like to thank Dr Doxiadis, The Foundation for Research in Childhood, NATO Science Council, and the Commission of the European Communities for inviting us to participate in this meeting. In WHO's regional strategy for Europe, we currently place great emphasis on health promotion, health care, and environmental issues in health. These are the three main objectives in our work, with the accent very much on preventive medicine. Ethical issues are of course of considerable importance in this field and this workshop will be of great value in furthering discussion.

MEDICAL ETHICS AND MORAL PHILOSOPHY

LUCIEN KARHAUSEN

COMMISSION OF THE EUROPEAN COMMUNITIES, LUXEMBOURG

DR CAMPBELL (CHAIRMAN)

It is now my pleasure to introduce Dr Lucien Karhausen who is an officer of the Commission of the European Communities, and is Deputy Director of the Directorate of Health and Safety in Luxembourg. Dr Karhausen has an MD from Brussels University and his specialities in medicine are internal medicine and epidemiology. He has the degree of Master of the Science of Hygiene from Harvard University and he has a continuing interest in the philosophy of medicine.

DR KARHAUSEN

In 1982 a committee was set up by the British Government to examine the social, ethical, and legal implications of recent and potential developments in the field of human assisted reproduction and the report, the so-called Warnock Report, was published in the middle of 1984.

One year after this first committee was established, the French Government set up an ethics committee with a broad brief to study moral problems raised by research in biology, medicine and health.

Both of these committees were composed of representatives of scientific, religious, legal, and lay viewpoints, but there is a major difference between them. The French Committee did not include any professional philosopher or ethicist, while the British Committee was chaired by the eminent philosopher and ethicist, Dame Mary Warnock.

Another interesting difference between them is that on the problem of surrogate motherhood, the French Committee reached clear, streamlined, and fairly definite conclusions. The conclusions of the British Committee were more sophisticated and provoked wide discussion. They made in fact two statements – a majority statement from 14 of the 16 committee members and a minority statement from the remaining two. After these reports came out, Professor Warnock underlined the fact that the minority report should not be underplayed or overlooked. The point I would like to emphasise from this is that the subject of medical ethics is not a chapter of law as the Council of Europe would like it to be. Nor is it a chapter of political science. It is not a chapter of medicine, it is a chapter of ethics.

David Hume in his Treatise on Human Nature, written in 1739, wrote a short paragraph which has been seminal and can perhaps be summarised by saying that one can never derive an 'ought' from an 'is'. The main issue is that there is a fundamental distinction between descriptive and prescriptive language. Science uses descriptive language, ethics uses prescriptive language, and one can never make an inference from descriptive to prescriptive language – in other words one can never make an inference from scientific statements to moral statements.

What does this mean in practical terms? Suppose I say that slavery is wrong and somebody asks me, why do you say so? There are two ways to answer that question. The first, which is akin to science, would be to make a survey of public opinion and see what the population thinks. An anthropologist might say I am against slavery because I have been brought up that way, that is my cultural background. Somebody else might say slaves are not paid for their labour and one cannot buy and sell people like cattle. But a slave merchant, and there are still slave merchants in the world today, might answer that he is aware of all of this and that he agrees with all these facts but that it does not follow from that that slavery is wrong.

The other way to answer the question, 'why is slavery wrong?', is the ethical way. This does not try to answer the question in terms of causes, in terms of determination, in terms of explanation, but in terms of grounds, in terms of justification, in terms of ethical principle.

I do not want to give you a definition of ethics. This would be beyond my own abilities and we would not have time to discuss that here. However, I would like to stress three major points.

The first is that ethical statements and ethical discourse are essentially prescriptive as we have already seen. The second point is that ethical statements should be able to be universalised. In other words, if one makes a recommendation which applies to one or two people or to a group, this recommendation, in order to be of an ethical nature, should be universalisable to all human beings, or at least to all human beings in a certain category, including the person who is offering the ethical statement. The third point is that ethical statements should be self-consistent, internally consistent. In other words, if we arrive at certain conclusions, they should be consistent with other ethical principles in the field and with generally accepted ethical principles in our society. This is perhaps one of the most difficult aspects of ethical conclusions.

At risk of over-simplifying, I would now like to divide ethical theories into two fundamental streams – first of all, the ethics of duty, deontological ethics, and secondly, the ethics of consequence, utilitarian ethics. The idea of ethics based on duty began with the thinking of Immanuel Kant. To the question 'why is slavery wrong?', the answer in this ethical approach is that slavery is wrong because it is wrong, and that is all. Why is killing wrong? – because it is wrong and that is all, that is the end. According to this view, we should consider not what the consequences of our actions are likely to be, but simply the conditions in which the act was performed.

Utilitarian ethics on the other hand takes a very different view. Here something is good if it is conducive to the maximisation of pleasure or happiness. Utilitarianism identifies moral good with the greatest happiness of the greatest number; we should act so as to bring the greatest good possible.

These two approaches are very closely linked again to two different streams in the field of medicine and health care. The doctor/patient relationship is based on the Hippocratic approach to disease, related to a deontological ethic. The doctor is entrusted to give care to individuals and his responsibility is the result of a contract between himself and the patient. Medical care is closely allied to the concepts of responsibility and duty, duties and rights. The patient has rights and the doctor has duties. Medicine is conducted under the god Aesculapius one of whose daughters was

Hygeia, the goddess of hygiene – you can see her beautiful head in the National Archaeological Museum of Athens.

Public health takes a very different approach. It is forward looking, it is concerned with populations, not with individuals; it is involved in laws, rules, organisations, and programmes. Its motives are welfare, prevention, cost allocation and its ethics are basically utilitarian.

These two streams in medicine can be exemplified in various ways and for those of you who are epidemiologists, I could just mention two types of indices, the attributable and the relative indices – attributable risk, relative risk, attributable effectiveness, relative effectiveness, attributable safety, relative safety. The point is that relative indices are helpful in order to identify causal relationships and those who are most directly involved in causal relationships are clinicians and clinical investigators. Public health officers are much more interested in size of population, how many people are going to be affected by a given health-care decision, so they are more interested in the attributable indices.

The conflict between these two approaches to ethics is continuously present in daily problems of health care. Medical researchers discover that private and public funds are much easier to obtain if they work on cancer than if they are interested in rare disease or even less newsworthy conditions like muscular dystrophy. Health policy-makers have a strong tendency to concentrate their efforts on disease and ailments which have a high prevalence. The problems of resource allocation in periods of scarcity result from the conflict between the ethics of duty and the ethics of utility.

I claimed earlier that medical ethics is a chapter of ethics, not of medicine. This does not exclude the importance of medical science and of the various disciplines which are and should be associated with medical ethical decisions. There is no doubt that in many cases theologians, priests, union representatives, should have their say. In other words, if medical ethics is a chapter of ethics and not of medicine, this does not mean that medicine, social science, economics, religion, or politics should be kept out. Medicine is of course, highly relevant to medical ethics but so are economics and sociology and public opinion. People's preferences must be taken into account in medical ethical decisions which after all concern people.

This brings us to the present meeting to its substance, its content, and its aims. Practical morality in daily life as well as in medicine is the result of a constant tension between what could be called conduct as opposed to ethics. Between the 'ought' and the 'is', there exist various more or less stable combinations which are interwoven into the fabric of life. There was a great distance between Greek behaviour at the time of Aristotle and what Aristotle was teaching in Nichomachean ethics and an incredible gap between Kant's Metaphysic of Morals and the teachings of Sigmund Freud. Our moral decisions, those which will be the focus of our discussions here, are and will be an effort to span the logical space, the unbridgeable gap between what we ought to do and what we actually do.

Philosophy teaches us that ethical propositions are neither true nor false, but human decisions and actions can be right or wrong, bad or good. Ethical philosophy is not going to give us an unequivocal answer to our moral questions, such as would be the case in logic, in mathematics or in physical science. Ethical philosphy is merely going to help us to clarify the issues, to help us to make consistent decisions and principled choices; it should help us also to disagree and to know why we may disagree; and it should help us to communicate. In the field of medical ethics, the ethicist is like the conductor of the orchestra. He may know one instrument, but he does not make music, he merely helps musicians to make music together.

DISCUSSION

Discussants: Campbell (Chairman), Beauchamp, Crawshaw, Gorovitz, Jeanneret, Knox, Martin, Pinet, Riis, Roy, Strasser, Tognoni, Trihopoulos, Veatch, Violaki

The basic issues for discussion throughout this paper concerned the whole approach to the discipline of ethics and three particular issues were highlighted. The first was the distinction between descriptive language, the language of 'is' and prescriptive or evaluative language, the language of 'ought'. The second was the assertion that medical ethics is a branch of ethics not medicine. The third was the question of whether ethical theories are based on an ethic of duty, a deontological approach, or an ethic of consequence, a utilitarian approach, especially in relation to public health issues.

On the first issue, discussion opened with a plea that the validity of the distinction between prescriptive and descriptive language be rigorously explored. David Hume made this radical distinction but it led him to put ethical statements into a largely emotive character, taking away any rational justification for statements in ethics. Some philosophers would want to say that we can have a science of ethics although the science has different rules from, for example, physics or anatomy.

In this workshop we are dealing with the question of health much as Plato dealt with justice and like him we should be prepared to take time to get our definitions clear and reject any pressure to dispose of such fundamentally important issues in too great a hurry. One way forward might be to widen the terminology from medical ethics to health care ethics.

The distinction between 'is' and 'ought' is by no means a clear one. The science of medicine is descriptive but it is also prescriptive. In public health, for example, if we say that immunisation against yellow fever is good, we are making a prescriptive statement. But we arrived at this prescriptive statement by an analytical and descriptive route. Ethics are open to scientific analysis, and if we agree that they can be analysed, we are getting into descriptive waters. There is much overlap between is and ought and we should beware of making too categorical a distinction.

On the point that ethical principles should be universalisable, a note of caution was also sounded. The idea of universal principles is attractive but almost impossible to achieve and in practice we should not opt too heavily for universality.

There are many traditional categories of philosophical and ethical thought according to which moral judgments are matters of demonstrable fact. These would range from the views of Kant who provided what he considered to be a logical rationale or justification to demonstrate a moral conclusion to theologically based ethics which in a very different way hold moral judgments to be matters of fact.

On the same issue, there are two very different questions that have been raised and which must be clearly distinguished from each other. One is the question of the gap between an ethical judgment and actual behaviour. We are all familiar with that gap and the practical problem of how to close it when it is clear what ought to be done but not how to get people to do it. This is the problem of how to induce moral behaviour and it is not a problem of ethics.

The other question, which is ethically much more interesting, is that of determining what is right and what is wrong. The kind of issues in preventive medicine that are ethically most challenging are those where we do not have a settled judgment about what is the right mode of behaviour. This should be the focus of our ethical concern – to clarify what are the problems and what the limits on preventive interventions.

On the second main issue – the assertion that medical ethics is a chapter of ethics not medicine – the borders of the subjects are not as clear or as tidy as such a statement suggests. There are so many problems in preventive medicine where both medicine and ethics are involved but where other factors like religious convictions and public opinion may also be very strongly implicated – abortion provides a clear example of this.

Medicine, as it is practised today, is full of value judgments. And medicine, without contact with philosophers, will end up in isolation, acting upon these value judgments which are often accepted without examination. In the same way, ethics must be open to interaction and cooperation with other disciplines which provide the raw material for its work. Medical ethics is surely medicine and ethics, both are necessary, neither is sufficient, and whenever the two work together something can be achieved.

It is important also, in considering the relationship of ethics to medicine, not to make the tent of ethics so large that it covers more than it is able clearly to contemplate. Many of the problems of preventive medicine are not narrowly medical. They are problems of the relationship of the citizen to the state, they are problems of the scope of government.

There are some who believe that ethics reaches that far and encompasses the task and scope of government. A kind of imperial quality can sometimes be detected in both medicine and ethics. But the relationship of the individual to the state and to government is a somewhat different problem from the duty of the physician to the patient, and we must try to keep the distinction clear in discussion. We must also take into account the other professions who make a contribution to preventive action.

It may be that the use of the term bioethics, largely used in the American and Canadian literature, could help in bridging the gap between medicine as a science and ethics.

On the third main issue raised in this paper – the distinction between the deontological and utilitarian approaches to ethics, there is a fundamental difference between ethics in therapeutic medicine where we are very much concerned with individual rights and ethics in preventive medicine where the population-based nature of the subject indicates that we are dealing with collective rights. Thus in preventive medicine we are more closely identified with the utilitarian approach to ethics.

Even this, however, is open to question. The core of the Hippocratic tradition in therapeutic medicine is that the physician will benefit the patient and protect him from harm – *primum non nocere*. To some, this is pure consequentialism. And although it is correct to say that ethics in public health and preventive medicine has been utilitarian in its approach thus far, it does not follow that it need be in the future. Any system of public health that emphasises justice and fairness rather than simple aggregate consequences would shift the ethic into an ethic of duty. Since preventive medicine can take place both at the level of the individual patient and in public policy for populations, we must allow the possibility of both types of ethical approaches at both these levels of preventive activity.

The central ethical conflict can be well illustrated by an example which does not involve personal morals – the question as to whether vaccination against measles should be compulsory or not. Some people would say it is right to make it compulsory because it prevents measles; others would say it was wrong because it was compulsory. To what grounds do we appeal to resolve this conflict? We have one set of opinions one way and one another. Are there any grounds for decision? Is it a question of majority? Is it a question of power – of one group over-riding another? Is it outside the field of ethics or is it an ethical problem ? This kind of issue is very difficult, very central, and must be addressed.

Much is known about how to improve health. One of the barriers to improving health by the application of that knowledge is our respect for individual choice and individual rights. One of the central issues in prevention is the determination of the constraints that limit what we can impose on people in the interests of their health. The example of compulsory vaccination is just one instance of a much broader category. We see people engaging in types of behaviour or refraining from engaging in types of behaviour that constitute life style choices detrimental to their health. If we want to maximise disease prevention, we have to minimise individual liberty – that is the heart of the ethical conflict and it is that conflict we must address.

The matter of majority rule is one which is regarded by some ethicists at least as some kind of arbitrary imposition. But it should be remembered that there is a tradition of political philosophy which believes that the majority has a rightful role in making determinations about what is called the common interest or the common good. In a very famous vaccination case in the Supreme Court of the United States around 1905, where a citizen was resisting vaccination, it was ruled that it was the duty of the legislator and the majority to determine what is in the interest of the common good and what is for the common benefit. That is a kind of answer to a very powerful question. Both are established in the western democratic tradition – we have a right to ask and we must try to answer. We must also try to be pragmatic rather than too theoretical in our endeavours to resolve the conflict. Otherwise we may run aground on the rocks of varying and irreconcilable philosophies and religious beliefs.

CONCLUDING REMARKS

DR KARHAUSEN

In conclusion, may I say a further word about 'is' and 'ought'. I was starting from a clear principle of logic – that from a set of descriptive statements, one can never derive a prescriptive statement, unless at least one of the premisses is prescriptive. When we say that science is written in a descriptive language, we think mainly of paradigmatic sciences, such as physics. There is no doubt that medicine is not a pure science and that it contains a prescriptive element. Why should we treat people ? The simple fact that we make a distinction between normal and pathological is already a value judgment.

My statement about where medical ethics belongs was made in a slightly provocative way to stimulate discussion. But there is a tendency, mainly in Continental Europe, to collapse into either medicine or law the space which should be devoted to medical ethics and I think this tendency must be resisted. What we must continue to strive for is a way to lay the foundations for a sound approach to ethics in preventive medicine.

EVOLUTION AND MUTATION IN MEDICAL ETHICS

G R DUNSTAN

DEPARTMENT OF THEOLOGY, UNIVERSITY OF EXETER, EXETER

PROFESSOR TRIHOPOULOS (CHAIRMAN)

It gives me great pleasure to introduce the first speaker of Session II, Professor Gordon Dunstan. Professor Dunstan is Professor Emeritus of Moral and Social Theology in the University of London and an Honorary Research Fellow in the University of Exeter.

PROFESSOR DUNSTAN

Before I begin my paper, may I express our thanks to Dr Doxiadis and his colleagues for their invitation to this gathering and for all the arrangements made for our comfort which are greatly appreciated. When I arrived at Athens Airport, I looked around instinctively for the welcoming chorus and the garlanded bull. I found instead the modern secular equivalent, two very friendly men with a minibus. The spirit was the same, one of xenophilia, but the means perhaps more efficient. I thank you very much for your kindness to us and for making us so comfortable.

Those who have followed the sequence of our papers will have noticed a change in my title. I was first asked to write about evolution in medical ethics and to deal with contemporary matters. After thought, however, it seemed to me to be important to ask what prompted each step in the evolution of our modern thinking about medical ethics and therefore to accept the notion of mutation, the trigger or spring which caused the development to happen. So I changed my title to 'evolution and mutation in medical ethics' and I shall try to concentrate on these mutations. Why did these developments in medical ethics happen?

The first reason was the emergence of a new science base for the art of medicine. Hippocratic medicine was grounded in observation and sound knowledge, and was especially opposed to the speculative theories of philosophers and the religious. A new knowledge base yields a new technology and new opportunities for intervention; so an ethics – a determination of right professional conduct – has to be formed in relation to these new possibilities and the new duties they imply. This present generation has seen most spectacular advances in knowledge and technology and therefore new opportunities for medical intervention, new challenges for ethical decision; and these ethical decisions must be worked out of a tradition of ethics which is very old and very live. Ethical thinking must be grounded in the relevant empirical facts: philosophical speculation or religious assertion not so grounded is useless to the practice of medicine.

The second factor causing mutation is response to external threats. The emergence of totalitarian political systems at about the same time as the knowledge base was increasing so rapidly caused an abuse of new knowledge and a corruption of professional practice. In reaction to this we were given the Nuremberg Code and the codes and declarations which have followed it from the World Medical Association and other bodies. The threat is not past. It persists, partly under authoritarian political regimes, partly wherever bureaucratic power or uncontrolled commercial advantage prevail, and partly when zeal for reputation drives someone more quickly or further than he ought to go, with a threat to human integrity. There the ethical defences must be raised.

A third factor is the upsurge of ideological fashion. One such now threatens to overwhelm the traditional concepts of duty and liberty with a new concept – or a newly-extended concept – of rights. This language of rights, though necessary in some contexts, becomes the more dangerous when it is exploited by consumerism and in legal systems in which the size of damages awarded by the courts determines the size of the reward for the professional lawyer, the contingency fee. So the language of medical ethics undergoes change, and the practice of medical ethics changes with it. It becomes a matter of contest, of conflicting rights, rather than a calm determination of duties in respect of people's interests and their liberties. To this I shall return.

Next comes the concept of health care. Municipal health services are very old in the Greek and Arab traditions. But we are now dealing with the concept of health services organised on a national basis, either by government as is the case in the United Kingdom with the National Health Service, or by commercial organisations with commercial insurance to pay for it. The result of this is a wide extension of the issues called ethical but which are complicated by economic, political, and social factors, extraneous to the practice of medicine but now involved within it. Problems of resource allocation, for example, are basically economic matters – a function of the gap between the wealth produced in the particular society and what is required to meet new medical health care needs. When there is a shortfall and supplies are limited, the question of how to allocate resources among conflicting disciplines arises – an essentially political question. The problem is basically economic and political; the ethical questions arise secondarily, as when clinical services are limited by restricted resources.

Next I take ethics in research. The change from mere observation to systematic investigation is fundamental. When we design research procedures to gather and assess knowledge in a controlled manner, capable more or less of objective assessment, a new method is introduced, with considerable ethical consequences, and this is a marked feature of our times. There is need of an ethics to control research and of institutions to maintain that control or supervision of research. (The Declaration of Helsinki, 1964, (revised 1975 and 1983) outlined the basic principles and rules. As we have already heard from Dr Karhausen's comments on the Warnock Report, we in the United Kingdom are trying now to devise institutions to supervise and oversee – not I hope to control by political means – the conduct of medical research in relation to early embryology, *in vitro* fertilisation and embryo replacement.) The need for such an ethics was made clear by abuses of research which took place, and not only in the totalitarian regimes. So we have seen the emergence of codes and institutions and research ethics committees, all a product of our time.

But questions still arise in the interpretation of the codes and the guaranteeing on the one hand of essential freedom for the pursuit of scientific knowledge and on the other hand of the essential protection of the integrity of patients and research subjects. Dr Richard Nicholson, who is here, has spent the last two to three years studying the codes of ethics with regard to paediatric research and the conflicting concepts that arise – the blurred lines between therapeutic and non-therapeutic research, between consent and assent and proxy consent; the quality of consent obtainable from children; and the legal anomalies that attend these questions. Similar questions will arise in all areas of research and they are basically ethical in content.

There are also for consideration new directions, or mutations, concerning the protection we ought to accord to human life, particularly at the beginning and end of life, the two critical areas. We now have new embryology and a rapidly developing study genetics, with improved techniques for remedying infertility in some of its forms. What are our liberties and what our responsibilities in relation to the cleaving embryo? May we exploit its research potential or by attempting to do so are we violating a fundamental human interest? In the old tradition, exemplified by Aristotle in terms of formation and animation and continued virtually unbroken and with only occasional challenge throughout Western culture until the latter part of the nineteenth century, homicide was not incurred until the embryo was formed, *formatus effigatus animatus* – that is, from about 40 days onwards. Now absolutists of various sorts drive the concern back to the very beginning of life, to 'the moment of conception' as they say (as though there were such a 'moment'), with vast problems arising both in practice and in ethics. We have to work at this.

At the end of life, we have new techniques for life or organ support, coupled with advanced studies of the brain and the central nervous system and the processes attending the death or destruction of the brain at its various levels. These have required a new ethics concerning death and dying: when do the duties to the living give way to the duties owed to the dying and when do these give way to the duties owed to the dead? This is a significant point of mutation in ethics in our time. The general ethics were stated in the Declaration of Sydney, 1968.

I return to political duress because this constantly arises in new and recurring forms. The abuse of psychiatry in some countries led to the declaration of Hawaii in 1977, and this is a matter for continued international, professional, and ethical concern. Less noticed, but equally pressing, are the problems of doctors in countries where mutilation is part of the penal system and torture is used in interrogation. Here must emerge a horrible conflict of conscience for the doctor. To give professional assistance in the amputation or care of amputees goes against the code of the World Medical Association; to refuse such assistance not only exposes the doctor to political ostracism and the threat of personal punishment but also leaves the victim in less skilled hands. How can this dilemma be resolved in countries where these practices are apparently coming back into use?

Lastly I turn to the discipline of words and stress the need for strict scrutiny and discipline of words used in ethical discussion. We were all asked to be provocative in the presentation of our papers, and so I shall be. Earlier I mentioned the swamping of the old concept of duties and liberties by the new language of rights. In fact, very often we do not need the language of rights as a basis on which to recognise obligations. We have duties, for example, to the Acropolis: but you cannot say that the Acropolis has rights. We have duties towards animals because they are sensitive and feel pain as we do, but it is not necessary to invent a concept of animal rights to teach us those duties or to make us practice them. We may go much further with the language of 'interests', 'moral claims', 'wellbeing', all evocative of duties.

I believe that the extravagant use of the language of rights is a reaction to threat. The medical profession should ask itself very seriously why the patient population feels so much under threat that it must resort to a language, indeed a barrage, of rights to defend itself against doctors. The answer will be complex: it is by no means all the fault of the doctors. The language of rights is bound to introduce confrontation into an exercise which ought to be one of mutual understanding and cooperation.

Ethics is the science of mutual expectation and a genuine medical ethics will include an ethics of patient practice as well as one of medical practice, and these must respond the one to the other. If we continue to exploit the language of rights in a combative way we are doing no service to doctor or patient. We produce a defensive attitude in medicine and more litigiousness. And the more litigious we become, the further we depart from the fundamental dependence on trust upon which medical ethics and good medical practice must be founded.

There is, therefore, great danger in the multiplication of rights, the invention of more and more imaginary rights, the resort to the language of rights to support everything which anyone would like to have or which people think would be good for them to have. I suggest a careful scrutiny of our language, especially during this conference. Whenever we are tempted to use the word 'right' or to allege a supposed 'right', let us ask ourselves two questions. First, what is the ground of that right, on what reality does it stand ? Secondly, what is the true interest to be protected by that alleged right, and have we other means and another language – that of duty or obligation perhaps – in which we could express or protect that interest more effectively and more easily?

DISCUSSION

Discussants: Trihopoulos (Chairman), Blaney, Campbell, Canosa, Crawshaw, Doxiadis, Gorovitz, Jeanneret, Karhausen, Riis, Roy, Sand, Strasser, Terborgh-Dupuis, Tognoni, Veatch, Violaki, Zander

The theme of mutation and evolution in medical ethics provoked a great deal of discussion, and once again three main areas emerged – first, terminology and the discipline of words; secondly, the diversity of health care systems and values and the ethical difficulties these raise; and thirdly the whole question of rights.

Difficulties with terminology are inevitable in such a diverse and multidisciplinary group but definitions must be clear and must be examined. The idea of having a glossary of terms used was suggested. Without this it was felt that there might be a danger of people talking about quite different things under the protection of terminology which has not been clearly defined.

One of the main problems with terminology in the workshop is likely to centre on the term medical ethics. The word medical has a wide range of applications but it is usually intended to mean medicine in the sense of the individual doctor-patient relationship. There is still a great reluctance on the part of many people to accept that medicine includes public health, preventive medicine, and the whole concept of promoting self-responsibility for health and healthy life-styles.

The importance of the discipline of words was emphasised. In an international meeting such as this, with representatives from many different countries and disciplines, it is often assumed that the main problem is the disagreement of words. We have, however, much more to fear from pseudo-agreement on terms which may mask completely different meanings and usages. Expressions such as autonomy, paternalism, informed consent are much used in the medical world. They represent complex and difficult concepts and must be properly scrutinised and defined before we simply transfer them into the context of health care ethics. Informed consent, for example, takes on a different meaning in the context of a programme of preventive action or research in a population rather than in the individual doctor-patient consultation.

There was discussion also on the use of the terms evolution and mutation. In the literature of the philosophy of science, dating from the writings of Kuhn, Lakatos, and Musgrave, the technical term used is revolution. Science is currently the most de-stabilising agent in our culture and what we are dealing with is in fact a revolution based on science.

We must beware of confusing medical ethics with something very different - the ethics of medical professionals, particularly as articulated in their codes, declarations, and organised writings.

The thesis that the emergence of new perspectives and new technology is a recent addition to the practice of organised medicine, with ethical consequences, is completely correct. But we must recognise that there are many different systems of medical ethics in the world, deriving not only from organised medicine but from various religious traditions and systems of political philosophy.

Virtually everyone writing in medical ethics in the United States in the 1970s, for example, was trained either in religious ethics or in liberal political philosophy. To the extent that those medical ethical traditions are the source of some of Professor Dunstan's comments, they represent not a mutation in medical ethics but rather the very interesting convergence of different medical ethical systems, in particular the tension between the long history of Christian medical ethics on the one hand and the Hippocratic medical system on the other. Viewed from this perspective, it is wrong to describe what is happening as a mutation. It is rather the interaction of different and potentially conflicting systems. The medical ethics described in this paper is certainly as old as the religious and philosophical traditions it represents. But it is true that ethical systems are different and one of the real challenges for medicine today is that physicians are being asked to choose between the ethics of the Hippocratic tradition and those of various religious traditions. To view this as a mutation of medical ethics seems to misread important historical tradition.

This leads on to the second main issue for discussion, the existence of so many different value systems concerning health care and so many different aspects of health even within one system. What does this mean for governments, what is their task, and how far are they supposed to go in trying to equate or balance these systems and aspects to provide effective health care?

This point was amplified in the international context by the example of a discussion on ethical aspects in perinatal medicine during a CIOMS meeting in Athens in late 1984. A Chinese doctor, living and working in China, had spoken of the policy of the one-child family in practice. There are areas of the country where at the end of the first year of life, the proportion of boys to girls is five to one with the clear implication that newborn girls are being killed. This chilling example shows how ethical decisions depend very much on a variety of factors including political pressure and economic considerations. Ethics in general should have universalisability as one of its main elements but in practice, the complexity of the subject and of the very different systems under which it has to operate must make that an unlikely goal.

Religion was mentioned as another very powerful force in the development or non-development of medical ethics, especially in countries, such as Spain, where religious belief remains at the centre of society. Physicians in this context are not free in many cases to make their own ethical decisions on such matters as abortion. Another element of importance in ethics is also the environment and our duties to preserve and protect the quality of this.

Economic matters were among those cited as external to medical practice but commonly involved in discussions of medical ethics. It is likely to be unavoidable henceforth for discussions about health policy and preventive medicine, and even discussions about treatment choices in individual physician-patient relationships, to acknowledge the significance of economic dimensions of health care. We can no longer sharply separate economic issues from the medical agenda. They are an inherent part of the complex array of factors that physicians and policy-makers must confront. Indeed some of the most difficult ethical issues involved in medical practice and health policy have been in precisely this area.

Ethical codes of practice can help to plot a route through the jungle of health care systems and values, and much attention has been paid to codes in relation to experiments and various kinds of clinical practice. But medical ethics can never be limited to the content of codes. Indeed it is a permanent state of the discipline that much of what medical ethics must be concerned about is what happens when the codes do not provide the answer.

Medical ethics is an enquiry into the principles that should underlie the judgments that have to be made by physicians, by policy-makers, by patients, when the codes do not provide guidance. It is impossible to cover all possible cases by the development of codes of practice. The capacity of events to unfold at a more rapid rate than we can develop collective wisdom about how to act means that codes will always be running behind the need to make informed and well-based judgments about what to do.

The question of rights was the third main area of discussion and a note of caution was sounded about abandoning the language of rights. This has become a language of common appeal beyond the restrictions of individual religious conviction. It would also be wrong to imply that only those who can be shown to have obligations are permitted to have rights – in any society there are bound to be groups of individuals who may be unable to meet any obligations but must be regarded as having rights. There was also felt to be need for more comment in this paper on the rights of parents and their children, sometimes a matter of conflict.

In an example from the State of Oregon in the United States, which will be described more fully in Session III, the word right was examined in relation to health. The US Constitution provided the model in its statement that no one has a right to happiness but rather a right to the pursuit of happiness. Thus in the Oregon experiment, citizens are not considered to have a right to health but rather a right to the pursuit of health, which means that they have access to the social allocation of right, relative to how they treat themselves.

Patients' rights movements are often attributed to a breakdown of trust and communication between patients and the medical profession, and dialogue and collaboration are much to be preferred to this kind of conflict. However, two questions arise. How do we influence doctors and other health professionals to try to promote better communication, and how can we alleviate the mistrust that is already established?

The rights of the receivers of medical care are absolutely central to the practice of medicine, and an emphasis on patients' rights becomes a very important ingredient in the development of a more ethically responsive approach by the health professions.

CONCLUDING REMARKS

PROFESSOR DUNSTAN

With many of the general comments made I agree because of course they were assumed when I wrote my paper. The paper took the shape that it did, because I tried to be faithful to what I was asked to do. And since I was asked to talk about evolution in medical ethics in the modern context I had to decide how to treat this material. I could simply have recited the contents of the codes and declarations one by one but, as we are all aware, this would have been a completely wasted exercise. So I had, in the best Aristotelian sense, to decide the form in which to mould my material and I chose the metaphor of mutation as my agent. The mutation metaphor is not inept. I was concerned to ask what triggered particular changes within this modern period. I do not accept 'revolution' as the word for the particular process I described, however applicable it might be to health care in general. I sought to identify changes in environment which occasioned changes or developments in ethics; and, in biological metaphor, the correct name for these changes in evolution is 'mutation'.

I do not neglect religion. I am in fact a priest of the Church of England and religion is part of my being. But I have had to learn when dealing with medical ethics to keep my religion under discipline and to decide when it is relevant and when it is not. I think it is a fair comment to say that I do not put the Hippocratic tradition and Christianity in conflict. I have studied the matter historically a little and I am convinced that the Hippocratic tradition was developed, carried, and moulded into the modern world partly through the Arabs and partly through the Christians. This is well-documented and could be demonstrated. Thus I do not accept the divergence and conflict of 'ethical systems' suggested. As a matter of history, there were no 'ethical systems': the Hippocratic, Jewish, Christian, and Islamic traditions were combined pragmatically at different times and places.

I am from time to time driven to consider the effect of religion in today's evolution of ethics. On the whole, I find that at present religion is being restrictive rather than providing an incentive to change. Certainly, the social conscience of the Christian religion is much directed towards the poor, the underprivileged, and the developing world; and probably it is, in some of its more lively and intelligent manifestations, considering the effect of our medical interventions in those fields. But in relation to the rapid development of the science base of medicine, modern Christianity seems to be trying to apply the brakes rather than to offer positive guidance for the future evolution of the use of new knowledge.

I should like to expand a little on the point of whether information or trust is the basis for consent. Of course there must be information, but sufficient information as to give a ground of confidence in the practitioner. It would not be appropriate or responsible to give your patient – even an intelligent patient – who is not trained in the scientific disciplines, all the knowledge that you possess. He must be provided with significant knowledge, knowledge that is morally significant, and which will enable him to say yes or no to what you propose or advise. There must therefore be a selective basis to the knowledge that you impart, and the purpose of that selection must be a moral one, to enable him to give an honest consent to what you want to do. He will consent or refuse your proposal, not on the basis of the total biological or technological information underlying your diagnosis, your prognosis, and your prescription, nor indeed on your display of statistical knowledge of probable risk or benefit. His consent will be based rather on whether he believes that you and your colleagues will give him at least the best he can hope for and serve his interests best of all. He is going to commit himself to you not to an array of knowledge. That is why I say that information is relevant but it is not at the moment a factor in English law as a basis of medical practice, although a test case is awaiting appeal in the House of Lords. Informed consent therefore still rests on trust. (Since the Athens meeting, the House of Lords gave its judgment. It upheld the Court of Appeal's judgment that 'informed consent' is not the basis of the doctor-patient relationship in English law, while laying on doctors the duty of informing patients appropriately and sufficiently of the risks they may incur.)

Finally, on the issue of patients' rights, of collaboration versus conflict, I venture to suggest that we should get better medicine if we work collaboratively than if we work in opposition, in a constant confrontation of one group of people having rights against another. If we think that this is probably true, then we must choose means to promote and encourage this more positive approach. My theme here was partly prescriptive, and partly a prescriptive possibility. The particular point of the rights of parents and their children was not developed for want of time.

THEORETICAL BASIS OF DISEASE PREVENTION

ROGER BLANEY

THE QUEEN'S UNIVERSITY OF BELFAST, BELFAST

PROFESSOR TRIHOPOULOS (CHAIRMAN)

Our next speaker is Dr Roger Blaney, Senior Lecturer in the Institute of Clinical Sciences at The Queen's University of Belfast and an expert in health services planning and evaluation and related issues.

DR BLANEY

Our special contribution in this workshop is of course in examining the ethical aspects of preventive medicine or preventing ill health. Ethical discussions to date have usually been about clinical problems in medicine, and this can be illustrated by two news stories, currently taking press headlines in Britain. One of them concerned the question of surrogate motherhood with a lady who was paid £6000 to bear a child for someone else. The other involved a man who had been on renal dialysis for many years and who, for various reasons, was discharged from hospital in Oxford although he still required dialysis. Clinical issues such as these do receive massive publicity and they have been the subject of a great deal of discussion.

But we must ask the question what is the point of making these distinctions between clinical and preventive medicine – are the ethical problems not basically the same whether they relate to an individual or to a large population?

And the answer to our question would in theory be two-fold. If the ethical problems involved can be reduced to certain fundamental principles, such as personal freedom or human rights, it becomes less important to distinguish between individual and population and the answer can be 'yes'. But insofar as the question suggests that prevention and treatment are the same or at least similar, the answer becomes 'no'.

Both methods of disease control – that is, clinical treatment of currently ill patients and preventive medicine – appear to have common first level strategic objectives, the prevention of premature death and the improvement of health. Even at this level, however, these similarities prove on examination to be spurious. If we ask another question 'to prevent premature death in whom?', the difference becomes apparent. In clinical medicine, the task is to prevent premature death in this individual patient who is under care at the present time. In preventive medicine, the aim is to prevent premature death in whole groups of people, in populations.

From the clinical point of view, the individual patient is being treated perhaps to the exclusion of other patients and perhaps even at cost to other people, and this introduces the whole concept of priorities and choices.

Professional ethical codes, which stress the protection of the patient, often with great fervour, can be construed as a remnant of a historical commercial contract between the doctor and the patient. In that context a more appropriate word for confidentiality may have been secrecy since there was competition between doctors for patients and some of these medical 'ethical' codes may have been founded in that rather than in any pure desire to do right. This may seem provocative, critical, even destructive but my objective is to stress the entirely different approaches of clinical and preventive medicine and to urge that we bear these in mind and subject them to scrutiny.

To balance these remarks, it is of course equally important to stress that action taken at population level affecting a large number of people can also have ethically undesirable aspects and when we make large mistakes, with millions of people, the results are likely to be catastrophic.

Another important aspect of my particular theme is the responsibility to acknowledge that when we act for the 'common good', we run the risk of depriving individuals of their freedom. Social action at population or community level is more often taken by the state and it has more potential for evil and for abuse. And I would like to re-emphasise that clinical and preventive medicine are intrinsically different in a whole range of areas. The population or community is different from the sum of the individuals who make it up. Society has an ethos which is built into its institutions, rather than its individuals, so that, for example, in large bureaucratic organisations employing many thousands of people, the loss of one individual, even the top man, makes no real difference to the institution. It continues with its own ethos, with its own traditions, irrespective of individuals and their power. The state and the population are rather like that in many ways.

Another important aspect in any consideration of the theoretical basis for preventive medicine is models of disease causation which are clearly crucial to any efforts in prevention – if we wish to prevent disease we must seek to understand its cause. The most pure type of prevention is that which tackles the cause of the disease before the disease appears.

Some of these causal mechanisms are of great historical interest, especially the model which included the element of morals or evil-doing. This still exists, for example, in the field of alcohol abuse. In some people's minds the problem of alcoholism or the alcohol dependency syndrome is wrapped up with a kind of moral judgment about how a person controls or fails to control his or her life and this model can have a major effect on what society does about the prevention of alcohol abuse.

In the past, this moral approach has been used, for example, in relation to outbreaks of epidemic disease. When the great cholera outbreak swept over Europe in the nineteenth century, it reached Ireland in 1832. The Government's approach at that time, which is quite recent in our terms, was to declare a day of prayer when the nation would acknowledge that it had been sinful and ask that God might arrest this plague and chase away cholera. By the next outbreak of cholera in 1869, John Snow and Edwin Chadwick had illustrated quite conclusively in statistical terms that cases of cholera were very closely associated with poor sanitary conditions, particularly in London. The 'day of prayer' concept as an approach to cholera had completely disappeared only 30 years later and, although the organism had not been identified, it was now known that poor sanitary arrangements were the cause. As scientific knowledge progresses, therefore, the idea of moral responsibility for disease, although it still exists among certain populations, tends to regress.

Many of these models, of course, offer us strategies for disease prevention. And here we should perhaps distinguish between primary prevention and each subsequent stage of prevention when interventions become more and more clinical, and the two approaches begin to overlap. The example of a man-eating tiger molesting a small village can help to clarify the issues involved. True primary prevention would mean capturing or killing the animal before it had time to strike but this would entail a system of communication and surveillance not available to the small community. The next best approach would be a secure fence around the village but the villagers are so preoccupied with individual defence and with treating and transporting the wounded that they cannot plan such strategic preventive action. The tiger, therefore, continues to terrorise the village and claims many victims, especially among the very young and very old.

This kind of specific situation can tell us a great deal about how the whole mechanism of prevention works. This has to be emphasised because we tend so naturally to slip back into clinical medicine again, instead of trying to foresee and tackle the problem before it actually arises.

And here we have an interesting problem in language because the word prevention means acting before the problem has arisen at all. Strictly speaking, therefore, prevention does not apply to population screening methods where the technique is clinical but the approach is public health. In our discussions, we should bear that type of consideration in mind.

One of the major difficulties in prevention is that its results may not actually be seen or be measurable for considerable lengths of time – sometimes even a generation after the action was taken. Governments, therefore, are not highly motivated towards preventive action because their normal term of office is three years or six years. There are no votes in saving lives 10 or 20 years hence and this presents a great challenge for preventive medicine.

Finally, a word should be said about paternalism. Paternalism is a term rather like bureaucracy. It is usually derogatory but in reality, like everything else, it has its attractive as well as unattractive aspects. What after all is wrong with your father looking after you when you are not able to look after yourself? One of the things we have to examine is whether populations or governments are justified in passing legislation or compelling people to do things for their own good. We all acknowledge that it is important for governments to do things for other people's protection, society generally, or for the protection of your neighbour, but is a government justified in taking action to prevent you or constrain you, or your freedom, in order to reduce your health hazard risks. That is a central question.

DISCUSSION

Discussants: Trihopoulos (Chairman), Canosa, Dunstan, Jeanneret, Knox, Nicholson, Pinet, Pochin, Riis, Roy, Violaki, Zakopoulos

Discussion of Dr Blaney's presentation centred on three main issues – first, the contrast between clinical and preventive approaches to medicine, secondly, the underlying conflict between the need for data collection and for confidentiality to be properly observed, and thirdly, the transfer of benefit from one group to another. There was a brief comment also on the ambivalence of religion in relation to ethics illustrated by Dr Blaney's reference to days of prayer as a response to outbreaks of cholera. The 'day of prayer' technique represented two beliefs – one that a god exists responsible for everything that happens and two that, because this god is moral, whatever does happen is not his fault but ours. In the cholera example, man's sin must have occasioned the outbreak – a dogma of religion dictating a course of action.

On the first main issue, the danger of creating too sharp a contrast between clinical and preventive medicine was raised. In the context of ethics it can be argued that there is no difference of principle involved. Individual patients are often dealt with in a way that includes prevention. Treatment is often called prophylaxis but this is here defined as 'medical procedures carried out within the doctor-patient relationship to prevent disease' so it is really two aspects of the same problem.

Controlled trials run by clinicians often concern huge numbers of patients, and when there is a national of international consensus on the treatment principle, the numbers are similar to those dealt with in preventive medicine. Conversely, community initiatives of a preventive nature – for example, policy on haemophiliacs or identifying cases of rare kidney disease for dialysis – sometimes concern very few patients, almost to the extent of the press being able to identify individual patients.

In recent years, individual physicians have been more and more involved in public health action and public health practitioners in individual preventive measures. It may therefore be more productive to address the common basic principles in the ethical context.

A plea for clarification and exactness of terminology was made and in addition to public health, preventive medicine, and prophylaxis, there should be a place for the relatively new concept of community medicine.

The second main issue for discussion concerned the conflict between data collection and confidentiality. Prevention is based on data collected and assessed in order to allow appropriate action to be taken. And, because of new technology, massive amounts of information are available. In a study of low birth weight, for example, information on each mother's parity, family planning procedures, drug taking and consumption of alcohol and cigarettes will be sought. It is assumed that this information is confidential but the computer is then in a position to identify cases of alcoholism, drug addiction, and so on. This raises an acute ethical conflict on the legitimate use of data collected and stored in this way.

Data collection is of course essential to preventive medicine – without it there is no basis for planning health policy. In Europe there is currently a difficult conflict on this issue between those who seek to protect individual rights and those who carry out research. In cancer registry, for example, epidemiologists are currently concerned that laws on data protection should not prevent them from collecting necessary data on environment, working conditions, genetic background, personal habits. This is a central and very difficult ethical issue.

The problem of transfer of benefit was the third main topic of discussion. Most social policies outside medicine involve transferring benefit from one group to another – from the elderly to the young and so on. In preventive medicine the same mechanism is at work but we usually do harm as well as good and the people we harm are not the same people as those to whom we do good. This raises another ethical dilemma.

In some cases, it is a simple economic transfer of benefit. In the United Kingdom, for example, £300 million has been spent in the last 20 years on the prevention of cervical cancer. This has presumably saved lives although this does not show up in the statistics. There has, however, been a huge absorption of resources which might have been better spent elsewhere. Thus we have transferred a resource from somewhere which we cannot identify to spend on something else, in this case the prevention of cervical cancer. We have done good for some people and we have harmed other people by depriving them of these resources.

This point can also be illustrated in the case of screening for cancer of the breast. For every woman identified and given earlier treatment for breast cancer, eight other women have undergone a biopsy which they would not otherwise have had, with all the anxiety and trouble that entails. Difficult as it is to get a surgeon to accept that there is such a thing as an unnecessary biopsy, the fact remains that we have done harm to eight women for every one who has derived benefit.

In vaccination, in the old situation of smallpox vaccination and the current situation of whooping cough vaccination, we injure some children for the benefit of others. In the case of rubella, we benefit the children of the girls whom we vaccinate but we injure the children of those who do not come for vaccination – in the unvaccinated proportion of the population, the age at natural infection is delayed and there will therefore be a greater chance of contracting rubella during pregnancy. Once again there is a combination of good and harm.

There are many other examples of this transfer of benefit. In Tasmania, for instance, there was at one time a shortage of iodine in the water supply and a high incidence of congenital hypothyroidism. The solution taken was to put iodine into the bread and this greatly reduced the incidence of cretinism. However, it caused hyperthyroidism in adults who had adjusted to the previous situation.

On the purely economic level, it was suggested that there can be very variable expression of government's political will to enact preventive measures. This was illustrated by three recent examples from British legislation. The first example concerned legislation to introduce childproof containers for drugs. It has been estimated that introduction of these containers cost about £1000 per child life saved. Then there was the legislation requiring all agricultural tractors to have a hard top driving cab to reduce the likelihood of serious injury in the event of accidents. In that example, the cost per life saved was around £100 000. In the third example, about 10 years ago, a block of flats in East London collapsed after a gas explosion and legislation was introduced to change British building regulations. It has been estimated that this has probably cost in the region of £20 million per life saved. One international example which must represent very good value is an estimate of the cost to the World Health Organisation of eliminating smallpox – US$ 4 per life saved. There is therefore a fantastic range of expenditure in preventing individual deaths, many factors are involved, and it is again a question of the transfer of benefits.

In some cases also, if prevention means saving lives, it simply means postponing death. And in some specific conditions, it could involve postponing a death that could have taken place at very low cost, both in terms of finance and possibly of suffering, to have it take place later, after a long period of chronic illness and decline and enormous cost to individuals and society. This is not to argue that we should allow certain groups of people to die more rapidly because it is economically more attractive but to draw attention to a potentially very serious ethical conflict in preventive medicine.

The question of competing claims and transfer of resources is a vital one. The basic decision is fairly easy in concept – to use resources best in saving human life. In practice of course it is much more complex and the argument has been complicated by interpreting it in terms of the cost of a human life saved which is medically rather objectionable. The essential criterion must be to use resources in the most effective way medically, given the perhaps idealistic requirement that there is a beneficent government willing to devote resources saved from a relatively useless health activity to another more advantageous activity.

This whole question raises another closely related ethical problem – who decides in competing claims? It is relatively easy for a public health official to estimate how best to use existing resources in the preservation or promotion of health. But for the public some uses of resources may be much more acceptable than others, irrespective of the actual amount of benefit to health.

CONCLUDING REMARKS

DR BLANEY

I have made a note of the points raised and they will be extremely useful to me in developing the theme. The three main issues raised – the different approaches, or perhaps we should now say the common ground, of clinical and preventive medicine, the competing claims of data collection and confidentiality, and the transfer of benefits and determination of priorities – are perhaps three of the most important and difficult ethical issues in the health field today. We must seek to increase discussion and awareness of these issues in an attempt to find reasonable, practical, and acceptable solutions.

DEVELOPMENT OF PREVENTIVE MEDICINE AND HEALTH PROMOTION

A H M KERKHOFF

MUNICIPAL HEALTH DEPARTMENT, LEIDEN

PROFESSOR BEAUCHAMP (CHAIRMAN)

I would like to add my thanks to Dr Doxiadis for arranging this meeting in this wonderful city. I now have pleasure in introducing the first speaker of Session III, Dr Kerkhoff, who is Director of Public Health Services in Leiden. Dr Kerkhoff's main interests are in prevention and he serves as a member of the Prevention Fund, a committee formed to give financial support to scientific research in the field of preventive medicine.

DR KERKHOFF

I would like to begin by apologising, firstly for the forthcoming unethical torture of the English language, and secondly for the fact that I am not going to do what I ought to do and this is unethical too. My job was mainly to give a synopsis of the evolution of preventive medicine in public health. This approach, however, has its drawbacks, and I am going to deal with the subject in a slightly different way.

We are too often inclined to consider institutions and regulations from the past as insufficient or even silly, probably partly because we are judging them by our own modern standards. Certain mediaeval public health administration measures, for example, were considered quite satisfactory in their own context.

Now to my paper. The idea that an ounce of prevention is worth a pound of cure is one of very long standing. It would not be difficult, therefore, to present a long list of measures taken in the field of preventive medical care in the past. But it is open to question whether such a chronicle (which has been given several times already by others more qualified than myself) would really relate to the subject of this workshop. It seemed more fruitful to consider ways in which the history of prevention could offer some clues for a solution of the problems of preventive medicine today. An ethical approach to prevention and public health is to examine the acts of government rather than of individuals – to scrutinise political activity. The ethicist must consider the motives of the government and whether these are wrong or right, good or bad. First, therefore, he has to define the moral parameters and to this end he has to consider the actions of the government against the background of the possibilities available to that government for taking preventive action. An ethical approach would be: 'ought implies can'.

In this context it is important to consider to what extent the 'can' in the past has influenced the actions and measures of governments. Broadly speaking, such actions can be divided into two main groups. On the one hand, there is the medical technical ability to reduce the incidence or prevalence of diseases in the population, and on the other hand, there is the administrative capability necessary to make the measures effective. The first element must obviously be to gain an understanding of the nature of a disease and its causation. Effective preventive measures can be discovered by chance. More frequently, however, they are the result of deliberate and systematic research. This presupposes a workable medical theory which explains a maximum of phenomena with a minimum of hypotheses. For a long time humoral pathology was such a theory. Historically speaking, it may be seen as one of the major theories, as it governed medical thinking from the time of the early Greek philosophers up to the beginning of the nineteenth century. In essence, the theory was that the human body is a reflection of the surrounding cosmos, a microcosm in the middle of a macrocosm. The elements of the macrocosm – water, air, fire, and earth – are found in the human body as 'humours' – mucus, blood, black and yellow bile.

According to this theory, the humours should be present in their correct proportions and relationships. Illness was seen as a disturbance of the harmonious balance of the humours. This imbalance was caused by environmental influences on the human body, through the air breathed, the food consumed, and also by the weather and the climate with which man was so closely related. Even the causes of epidemic diseases could be explained by this theory – they resulted from pollution of the ambient air which could affect large groups of people at the same time (the so-called miasma or humoral theory). It is clear that this theory was very effective in disease prevention. It taught the importance of a good diet and a sensible way of life in general. It also explained why living in cold and humid places was unwholesome and why swamps had to be avoided.

The positive effect of this humoral theory is well illustrated by the extensive sanitary provisions in the cities of the Roman Empire and the numerous health regulations which were in force in the Middle Ages. In the Low Countries, for instance, it was forbidden to pollute the water upstream from a brewery. Even in the nineteenth century, this ancient theory was the main principle for the founders of modern public health, Jeremy Bentham and his disciples Thomas Southwood Smith and Edwin Chadwick.

What even this short diversion into history shows is that a medical theory – be it correct or not – is necessary to enable government to take preventive measures. But it can be demonstrated also that the decision to take preventive measures does not depend upon medical theory alone. On closer examination of the problem, we discover another phenomenon – namely, that government does not always apply the available knowledge. The sorry lot of the mineworkers in ancient Rome and of the mediaeval people without municipal rights provide examples where available medical theory was not applied, and we can conclude that government actions are not only or always based on the availability of a coherent medical philosophy. Apparently the decision to take preventive measures depends not only on the availability of a coherent medical philosophy. Let us, therefore, consider the need for an administration capable of executing preventive measures.

A good example here is provided by the 'Natural and Political Observations on the Bills of Mortality' of John Graunt, published in 1662. In seventeenth century England, mercantilism taught that the nation's prosperity can best be increased by a maximum export effort and the minimisation of imports. For a high level of exports, high production is necessary and this requires a healthy labour force, since sickness and poor health reduce productivity. In this context, political arithmetics were developed – something we would describe now as an epidemiological analysis of the state of health of a population. Graunt's observations suggested, for example, that gout and kidney stones were a constant percentage of causes of death while measles and typhus, by contrast, were not. Graunt also studied the differences in death rates in the inhabitants of towns and villages and, on the basis of this research, he strongly advocated collective preventive measures. The authorities were very much interested in his observations and advice, but lacked the organisational or administrative means to take effective measures.

From this example we may conclude that the existence of an effective administration is a necessary but not sufficient argument for a government to take preventive measures. We have only to think of scurvy for which an effective form of prevention was already known in the sixteenth century. It was, however, 250 years before the consumption of lime juice was made obligatory by the Royal Navy, this in spite of its status as an established and effective organisation. One possible explanation for this phenomenon is that the sailors were outside the political structure of their country and this might also explain why the slaves in the Roman mines were not cared for.

These examples seem to justify the conclusion that taking preventive measures is not the automatic result of the possibility of taking them. What is needed as well is a motive which is conditioned by existing economic, political, cultural, and ideological factors. This point of motive has been clearly described previously by George Rosen in the early 1950s and is supported by many examples from the recent history of preventive medicine. One of the best examples of political motivation is Bismarck's introduction of a social insurance system to steal a march on the socialist opposition. There are numerous examples of economic motivation, apart from the one already quoted, and even Adam Smith was not opposed to governmental involvement in preventive public health services. On the ideological side, the thoughts of Jeremy Bentham could be mentioned. He defended the greatest happiness of the greatest number of people as an aim for the government which included preventive health services.

In summary, the preventive actions of government in the past have not depended solely on the means available. Preventive measures were not the automatic result of the intrinsic merit of a particular preventive strategy. There must also be some type of motive. The criteria which carried the day in the end can only be identified by thorough historical research which places the preventive measures in their appropriate context.

The ethicist can profit from this historical research, especially if he does not restrict his observations to the field of moral and other motives but includes the tension between various ethical doctrines. After all I believe that it is this tension that confronts us in the health field today with some very difficult, painful, and intractable problems.

DISCUSSION

Discussants: Beauchamp (Chairman), Campbell, Dunstan, Gorovitz, Pochin, Roy, Strasser, Tatsis, Terborgh-Dupuis, Trihopoulos, Tognoni, Veatch

The main strands of discussion on Dr Kerkhoff's paper focussed on two central ethical conflicts – equity versus efficiency and individual freedom versus the public good.

The references to Adam Smith and Jeremy Bentham were the first point of comment. While it is true that their philosophies did support what might have appeared to be preventive health measures, the basis upon which they did so was quite restricted. There is the notion of a basically laisser faire kind of economic theory of the Adam Smith type where we pick up the obvious problems bequeathed by this, but do not make a wholehearted effort to ensure that governments take full responsibility for the welfare of citizens. In the case of Bentham, the problems with his particular form of utilitarianism are well known. This kind of simple utilitarianism can support only the crudest forms of readjustment of social disbenefit and cannot supply the kind of philosophy necessary for other kinds of health promotion and health prevention in society.

In his presentation, Dr Kerkhoff made the point that after we look at history, we must then consider appropriate contemporary arguments to support what we might now wish to see in the area of prevention and promotion of health. Neither Smith nor Bentham will do at this point. We must find some other kind of commonly shared philosophy which is much more positive in its support for notions of equity and equality. Perhaps some contemporary history should also be considered. What is the behaviour of physicians and philosophers tied to real cases? Consideration of some of the controversial issues in preventive medicine in different countries would be very valuable – as, for example, differing policies on psychiatry or on fluoridation of the water supply.

Space and attention must also be given to the fact that the development of the idea of prevention is not only a discussion of our growing sense of the role of the environment and causal factors, but also a changing and developing sense of our feeling of membership in the political community. The distinction made earlier between treatment and prevention, is, in the context of public health, nearly always discussed in terms of the individual and the population. The term population has a sort of scientific connotation. But we must also define it in the political context and examine what we mean by population here.

At precisely the time Chadwick, Smith and others were developing preventive measures throughout Europe and the United States, there was a growing sense of the national community and its responsibilities, and an increasing awareness of the relationship of citizens at the local level to that national community. And these social and political developments were just as important as the scientific changes. All the science in the world is impotent without a sense of membership of the national community. Without this it is impossible to involve people and seek their participation in preventive schemes, planned for the common good. So scientific developments must be balanced with political.

There is an important difference between the mid-nineteenth and mid-twentieth centuries in public health terms. At the time when public health measures were initially being introduced, the benefits from rather modest changes were so dramatic that no one needed to dwell on the difference between the greatest good for the greatest number, the Bentham principle on the one hand, and distributing benefits fairly on the other. Utilitarian principles, therefore, led us easily into preventive health measures.

In the late twentieth century circumstances are very different. Now it seems that we are being forced to choose between a preventive measure that will do the greatest good for the greatest number on the one hand, or an alternative preventive measure that will distribute benefits fairly. A particularly dramatic example of this from British literature is provided by an empirical cost-benefit, cost-effectiveness analysis study which demonstrated there are two ways of screening British schoolgirls for bacteriuria. One of these clearly found the most cases per pound invested and it would seem on Benthamite grounds to be the obvious choice. Only later was it discovered that the alternative method, which used a lot more professional nursing skill, distributed the finding of cases far more fairly. The first method found cases but found predominantly middle class cases, whereas the second method found cases more fairly across all social classes. This presents us with a difficult ethical choice. Do we want to be Benthamites and be efficient about it? Or do we want a more egalitarian distribution of benefits even if the method is less cost-effective and less efficient? That seems to be a critical valid choice for late twentieth century preventive medicine. In the mid-nineteenth century the choices were not nearly as subtle.

Another complicating factor here is that of time in the choice between equity and efficiency. There may be a system which is temporarily inequitable but is very efficient. It is unequal for the time being but within 10 years, it will provide equity in addition to efficiency. What is the decision here and what the time reference?

A further ethical problem for government in this area of distributive justice is the choice between developing centres of excellence or maintaining centres of routine service. This question of justice, especially distributive justice, is very often going to be the central ethical issue in this particular area of preventive medicine. The problem then confronts us that there are very few really good treatments of the philosophical problem of distributive justice. This is a genuinely new issue which has not been well aired within the field of health care ethics thus far, and we are therefore very much at a growing edge of discussion. We are also dealing with what has been described as an extralogical choice. In equity and efficiency we are trying to compare factors which are inherently mutually exclusive and our decision, therefore, will be either political or social but cannot be strictly logical.

Distributive justice is certainly one of the central ethical issues but it is not the only one which must be emphasised. Even if we are clear in making that extralogical choice – the policy decision about whether to choose more expensive equity or more efficient distribution – we still face the problem of the extent to which we respect individual liberty at the cost of public health. That is an issue that runs parallel to the problem of distributive justice.

When there are measures that we know will be conducive to the public health, do we impose them on those segments of the public that seek to resist such imposition? That is another example of a value conflict.

The example of screening schoolgirls for bacteriuria reveals two different values that are clearly in conflict with one another – the value of efficiency and the value of fairness – and this is a problem because we respect both of those values. The dilemma is how to decide in the context of conflict between two respected values. Similarly, we respect promotion of public health but also individual freedom of choice and the conflict between those two values is one of the central current dilemmas in preventive health. In the state of New York, for example, it has recently become illegal to drive a car without wearing a seat belt. In some western parts of the United States, the notion of such a law, would be completely unacceptable because it would be seen as a violation of individual liberty, regardless of the public health consequences. So there is an example in which we deal with the conflict differently in different contexts.

A possible way out of the conflict could be by trying to define criteria of what is good for man or for people. The philosophy of Warnock is relevant here in its assumption that we can know what is good for people as individuals and as a society. Once we know this, there is a way forward because the value which is best for people must prevail. This may be an attempt to find an anthropological answer to a moral question but it may help in reaching a solution.

This issue, the individual versus society, is perhaps the central problem of ethics in preventive medicine. But if we are looking for a clue to the understanding of the problem, we have to look at it from the societal point of view. In some societies, values may differ very markedly between the individual and the population on a particular issue. The example of the one child family in China is an illustration of this – viewed from the individual point of view this is clearly a coercive policy, but it has been accepted by Chinese society as a whole.

Differences in seat belt legislation in various American states highlight the problem of implementing health policies when there are different value systems within a particular society. The ethical dilemmas are much more acute in western pluralistic societies with conflicting value systems. But although the problems are certainly more acute in these circumstances, many of the difficulties arise from a conflict of values within us individually, not as particular groups such as the conservative religious right and the liberal secular left in the United States, or between Muslims and Jews, Catholics and Protestants. That kind of diversity obviously adds an extra dimension of difficulty but even within a homogeneous community, there remains the problem of how to allocate scarce resources, there is still the conflict that any individual feels between different values.

On the tension between individual liberty and public health, the question also arises as to whether it is affected by the type of health care system involved. Is that tension more acute in a system in which health care is fundamentally provided by public funds or in one in which it is privately funded?

To resolve the dilemma, to get the best results in respect of liberty, we need a method and a workable method might be in terms of presumption. In democratic society, we would begin with the presumption in favour of the liberty of the individual; we would rebutt that presumption when we reach the point of social need, overwhelming the individual's right to dissent. In authoritarian society, the presumption begins with the individual doing what the state decides.

A note of caution was sounded about using the same terms for so many different problems. Individual freedom applied, for example, to seat belts is quite different in its implications from individual freedom applied to vaccination. In a liberal society it is very hard to justify compulsory preventive health measures against the will of the individual when all these measures do is improve the health of the subject of the intervention. That is a pure violation of liberty. On the other hand, virtually everyone recognises the legitimacy of intervening, violating liberty, when there is a social need.

The critical question is which of the two criteria that we have been discussing should be used as the trigger point for determining that there is a social need. If, on the one hand, we use utilitarian criteria, then we can intervene whenever there is a net improvement in aggregate health statistics by intervening – a very easy justification for intervention.

The alternative is to say that we are justified in health promotion measures against the will of the individual only in those cases where the result is a more just distribution in society. That is a much more conservative justification for intervention and is very different from the intervention justified solely on the basis on improving aggregate health indicators.

CONCLUDING REMARKS

DR KERKHOFF

I am delighted that my contribution has evoked such a wealth of interesting discussion. Nevertheless, I am reminded of the verdict of the well-known American car manufacturer, Henry Ford, on the use of history – 'history is bunk'. We must examine critically the role of history in deepening our insight into ethical problems which confront us today.

PROFESSOR BEAUCHAMP

We certainly can and, I think, have learned useful lessons from history. But what we have been talking about here is a simple problem of democratic theory. In my own personal view, there is a conceit, largely found in the Anglo-Saxon countries, that democratic theory is liberal democratic theory with the presumption for the individual, and that the alternative is authoritarianism with the presumption for society. There is another very generous and large body of democratic theory that falls between these two approaches.

ETHICAL ASPECTS OF PUBLIC HEALTH LEGISLATION AND THE ROLE OF THE STATE

GENEVIEVE PINET

WORLD HEALTH ORGANISATION, REGIONAL OFFICE FOR EUROPE, COPENHAGEN

PROFESSOR BEAUCHAMP (CHAIRMAN)

Our next speaker is Dr Genevieve Pinet from the World Health Organisation in Europe. Dr Pinet is a lawyer by training and is active in WHO in the relationship between law and policy, and health promotion and disease prevention. Dr Pinet's paper will be followed by a short presentation by Dr Ralph Crawshaw from Oregon.

DR PINET

I was originally asked to speak on public health legislation and the role of the state in prevention. However, in the meantime, the title of my presentation has become 'Ethical aspects of public health legislation and the role of the state.' I hope this meeting will help in defining my subject and in discussing relevant examples from different countries.

I would like to start with two general remarks, one addressed primarily to the lawyers and the other to the physicians, remarks which may be useful in understanding the conceptual problems encountered by those dealing with the question of prevention and legislation in the health field. In reading the work of lawyers in this field, I have the impression that they are sometimes ill at ease in dealing with prevention because they are used to relying on clear-cut definitions and well-defined concepts. They tend to resent being confronted by several differing definitions which may seem too vague to the legal mind.

With regard to physicians, also, there is no unanimity on the meaning of prevention and differing definitions abound. This is due mainly to the evolution of the concept of health, notably to some of the uncertainties of its enlargement. It is certainly a good thing to be able to enlarge the concept of health, including new related health sectors, and to find new approaches, taking advantage of the progress of science and technology. There is a need to find some sort of unified approach.

First, by way of introduction, I would like to refer to the WHO constitution, and to quote from its preamble that 'governments have a responsibility for the health of their people which can be fulfilled only by the provision of adequate health and social measures.' The success of these measures often depends on the combined action of health legislation and health education. I would also like to mention the WHO concept of prevention which proposes three levels of application of preventive measures – primary, secondary, and tertiary.

I intend to illustrate the contribution that health legislation could make on these different aspects of prevention applied to the whole range of comprehensive care usually described under the following four categories of service: health promotion, health protection, health recovery through diagnosis and treatment, and rehabilitation.

Let us take first health protection. This is in fact primary prevention, prevention at its best, which aims to avoid the occurrence of illness and accident in a given population by acting on causes and risk factors. Here, during previous discussions, we have mentioned the intervention of law, with compulsory notification of certain types of disease and compulsory vaccinations. Smallpox eradication has also received comment and this is a most convincing example of the synergy between law and prevention. We can speculate too on the state of health of the world population without the WHO International Health Regulations, given the enormous and ever-increasing socioeconomic phenomenon of population movement on a global scale today. We also know that legislation has long provided support for various preventive health programmes, like occupational health, school health, road traffic accident control, and food control. This latter provides the most demonstrable example of the combined action of primary prevention and legislative measures at the national level, with international repercussions because of the increasing growth of trading in food products between countries and socio-cultural tourism.

If the chance offered by primary prevention has been missed, which means when illness or accident cannot be avoided, we appeal to the curative arm to restore health, and here secondary prevention may also be accomplished through early diagnosis and prompt treatment. Public health action in this context might include compulsory medical examinations for a particular disease or for high risk groups – for example, medical control of immigrants – through public health legislation. In terms of treatment, coercive action by law might be used to prevent spread of communicable diseases such as tuberculosis or sexually transmitted diseases.

Let us turn now to tertiary prevention where the main objective, after treatment has been applied, is to avoid further physical or psychological damage, particularly of an irreversible nature. The goal is to reduce incapacity and handicap, and above all to avoid loss of autonomy and prevent dependency upon the family and the community. In this respect, a particularly interesting group is the elderly. In this area of medical and social readaptation, legislation is needed to support the reintegration of people into society, to ensure that their rights are respected, and to avoid discrimination. Rehabilitative measures offer the opportunity not only of alleviating suffering for the individual but also of reducing the burden on society of supporting physically or mentally disabled patients. It is a challenging social issue but a very expensive one which can only be successfully promoted with the support of a strong legislation in the medico-social field, able to ensure equity in the distribution of resources.

There is nowadays increasing insistence on preventive action taking place at an earlier level, before health protection. Such measures are known as health promotion and here the health concept becomes more dynamic. The notion of wellbeing is transcended by the notion of quality of life. There are two main aspects to this approach which we can put in the health promotion category: protection of the environment and concern for lifestyle. This is not surprising when we consider that many modern illnesses – maladies de civilisation – have a mainly environmental and behavioural origin. It should be emphasised here that health promotion measures are an extension of primary prevention because they also depend on taking action against causal factors detrimental to health.

Let us consider first health promotion and the environment. Environmental factors conducive to health are well-known: they include making available safe water and sanitary facilities, suitable housing, adequate sports and recreation areas, efficient transport systems, measures for accident prevention. Health promotion also implies guarding against the danger to health caused by physical or chemical pollution, radioactivity, and noise. In this context, it is worth mentioning the efficient monitoring and substantial reduction in atmospheric and water pollution now being achieved in many industrial European countries. The encouraging progress in dealing with environmental health problems is undoubtedly the result of environmental health legislation enacted and implemented during the last decade. It reflects the importance of law as a tool in the quest for a better environment and improved public health. But it is also there that the most frightening threats to health may occur as we have seen in the industrial catastrophes in Bhopal, Seveso, and Mexico. This is a very cruel reminder of the necessity of strengthening legislation to give better protection for the populations living in these high-risk, industrialised areas. Transportation of potentially noxious products and disposal of radioactive waste with the least danger is another pressing environmental issue, to be regulated by governments. Countries have to rely on international environmental legislation to protect them.

Health promotion also involves efforts to increase physical, mental, and emotional wellbeing. One way to achieve this is by improving individual behaviour or influencing lifestyle choices. In terms of prevention this means avoiding harmful personal habits – using seatbelts, wearing helmets, adopting a sensible diet, limiting alcohol consumption, not smoking, taking physical exercise are examples of positive health-related choices. The important point is that the decisions taken are under the control of the individual who can intervene directly and decide personally on acceptable health risks, sometimes referred to as voluntary health risks.

Here we are entering the core of an ethical problem. To what extent, for instance, should society tolerate those personal health risk choices which appear to have dangerous implications for others? Has the individual the right to take a voluntary health risk? Do any voluntary health risks in fact exist, since we are all very much influenced by our genetic inheritance, education, social class, family background, religious beliefs? Can society intervene only when the individual presents a danger to others, as in communicable disease, alcoholism, or certain types of mental illness? Do we allow a certain degree of paternalism in such situations, as sometimes found in the wording of professional codes?

Why should society bear the burden of its citizens taking risks with their own health, particularly when many social security systems are obliged to pay the bill and when the limited resources may force a selection among patients or extend the waiting time for the treatment of someone else? Is health so valued in our society that a prevalent ideal of social justice would hold individuals responsible to the community for not being careful of their own health? Some may feel that if we go too far in this direction, there is a danger of victimisation of the sick by overstressing individual responsibility towards health. And governments might also be tempted to abandon some existing preventive health action. We could end up with a kind of medicalisation of society which would be almost the reverse of the original intention of the preventive action. Others may feel that in the realm of personal behaviour-related illness, society has the right to expect individuals to be responsible for their voluntary health risk choices which affect the health or financing of society. These are moral and ethical issues awaiting society's judgment.

Before concluding my presentation, I would like to say a brief word about the unprecedented achievements of research and the ethical implications these raise. Progress in biology and biotechnology brings ethical problems which are of great current concern in public health, in law, in government, and in society in general. Reference was made earlier to a recent controversy in a London hospital surrounding a surrogate mother. This is just one example of the problems that can arise from progress. A newborn baby was deprived of parental care from the first days of life because the law overruled parental love. Who considered the serious potential repercussions on the health and future emotional balance of the baby? Surely we should try to foresee such unacceptable situations, to take preventive action on a practical level, and to find a compromise between medicine and law and the expectations of modern society whose traditional values are changing profoundly.

To conclude, I personally am convinced, as is the World Health Organisation, that we have reached a turning point in prevention. Prevention has become a dynamic and evolving process, taking advantage of the new possibilities of biotechnology, the tools of modern epidemiology, the input of the social sciences, the resources of information technology, the techniques of the media and of health education, and the possibilities of health legislation. The resources are immense and have not yet been fully used.

SUBSIDIARY PRESENTATION

OREGON HEALTH DECISIONS

RALPH CRAWSHAW

2525 NW LOVEJOY, PORTLAND, OREGON

You have before you a paper entitled Oregon health decisions and the politics of bioethics. Since I assume you will not yet have had the opportunity to read this, I would like briefly to outline what I believe is an experiment in the realpolitik of bioethics. I hope I might stimulate some of you to try to duplicate such experience in your own communities in order to test its validity.

Oregon is a province, a state of the United States. It measures 500 x 650 km and it has a population of 2.5 million. We spend approximately $2.5 billion each year on health care and we have a health system that is out of control. I speak as Chairman of the State Health Advisory Planning Board. In that capacity I was struck over the years by the tremendous amount of human suffering which came to me informally. This suffering assaulted me because I had no way of responding to it. How do you respond, for example, to someone saying that they do not wish their grandfather to be kept on a life-support machine, that their county no longer has a public health department, or is it right for health care to be allocated on the basis of who knows the senator in charge of allocation? Given that kind of suffering and accusation, I found that there were a number of people within the community willing to address the problem of bioethics as bioethics. We were fearful in attempting this that we might be taken over by zealots, that the pro-life group or the end-stage renal dialysis group might wish to coopt what we were doing. This fear, as it turned out, was groundless.

Government was not interested in participating and so in order to carry out the project, we had to raise the money independently. One of the ironies of this was that the health planning system, a number of whose employees we wished to involve, could only cooperate in return for reimbursement. So we had to pay government to pay attention. In the end we paid about $18 000 to government to pay attention to people's problems with bioethics.

We have a health planning system that divides the state up into three areas. We asked each area to find citizens interested in bioethical experiences. These came mainly from those who had suffered from the existing system in some way – those, for example, with a retarded child not considered eligible for care at the state hospital but not eligible either for care at home; people caught in the bureaucratic vagaries of the system.

We took a cadre of 45 people and brought them to Portland, Oregon in 1982. We also brought members of the President's Commission on the Study of Bioethics to Portland as faculty and for two days we trained the 45 local people in the discussion, the language, and the experience of bioethics in health. Some of them attended hospices, some went to neonatal centres, but they all came close to the problems involved. We recorded this experience on a video cassette which shows the experiences of ordinary people brought up against the problem of trying to understand who should be in control of a system that is out of control. We provided our group with a great deal of information. It was then their task to go out into the community and to begin to educate our 2.5 million people. They succeeded in gathering together 5000 individuals in 300 different meetings. These meetings generally started with a discussion based on the cassette, which provided some sort of language to begin with, and the usual opening remark was how come doctors make so much money! The crew was trained so that they did not stop at that point but progressed to some of the other issues.

We also formed a cadre of four advisory boards. The solons of the professions of medicine, nursing, law, and religion in the state were asked to donate their time and reviewed all the material in order to refine and validate it from a professional point of view. They also served as speakers who met for discussion and then conducted the meetings.

As a result of this exercise, we asked for feedback on the various problems that people felt they were facing in their health care delivery system. About 1000 responses were received from people on issues that they considered particularly important. We collated this material and in October 1984 held a People's Parliament to which each section of the state sent a specified number of delegates. There were teachers, bankers, journalists, doctors. We spent an entire day in which we took resolutions that came from the community and began the debate as to what our health value system should be in Oregon. We have 45 resolutions which are currently being published.

Among the factors that emerged as important were autonomy, social allocation, prevention, justice (with particular reference to malpractice). We had a tremendous response in terms of concern about children and the idea of prevention through neonatal services proved to be a real underlying concern. The other major concern was the prolongation of life without quality. People wanted their elderly and suffering parents disconnected from life-support machines yet could not achieve this.

We have solved the question of autonomy, at least partially. If you wish to live a destructive life, you are free to do so, but you should pay the price. If you want to ride around without a helmet on a motorcycle, you should be charged the full cost of caring for all the people who have injuries as a result. Cigarette tax, we proposed, should be raised 88 cents a pack because that is what it costs to take care of the resultant emphysema. If you wish to smoke it is your choice, but you should pay the price which is considerable. We are very much interested in increased education at high school level on death and dying. We believe that our communities do not understand the whole process of death, or indeed reproduction, as biological experiences.

In conclusion, may I say that I think our problem is that we are experts without a forum. And that is what should be built – forums throughout the world where people can develop their health values in the Greek tradition.

DISCUSSION

Dicussants: Beauchamp (Chairman), Blaney, Campbell, Canosa, Dunstan, Gorovitz, Knox, Martin, Roy, Strasser, Tognoni, Veatch, Zakopoulos

Discussion on Dr Pinet's paper and Dr Crawshaw's short presentation centred on two main issues – the role of the state and the right to health.

On the role of the state it was suggested that it might be useful to distinguish various different ways in which the state can act in respect to preventive measures. These should be distinguished because they have very different consequences.

One way is, of course, to take coercive measures as discussed earlier. The state can require behaviour like wearing a seat belt while driving and it can forbid certain types of behaviour.

The state can have an educative role. A government, without infringing individual liberty in any way, can engage in a campaign of public education that relies on the judgment of individuals, voluntarily, to make changes in how they live.

The state can also provide incentives without coercion through tax benefits, or by influencing the way in which insurance rates are structured. That is another kind of role that is much milder than coercion – persuasion might best describe it.

Some government action limits the liberty of individuals not for their own benefit but for that of others. So, for example, when it is forbidden to sell certain food products, it is not the consumer's liberty that is restricted so much as the liberty of producers or suppliers. That is a different kind of restriction, often called indirect paternalism.

Government can also facilitate activity. The exciting tale from Oregon describes an activity that arose not from government action but from a coalition of like-minded independent private forces. But a government could undertake to facilitate a similar process in the interest of public health.

Thus, when we talk about the role of the state, we must bear in mind the great diversity of activities that a state undertakes in the interest of pursuing public health. There seems also to be a natural tension between people who are interested in preventive health on the one hand and the state on the other. This natural tension, the health people would suggest, is due to the reluctance of the state to take on the role of being a health provider or protector. A very good example of this exists in the United Kingdom. A few years ago the British Government set up a think-tank on the alcohol problem. This was a group of civil servants who looked into the problem of alcoholism in the UK and produced an extensive report. Not only would the Government not accept the report, it was in fact suppressed. As many of us know, the document was eventually smuggled out of the United Kingdom and published in Sweden where it is now available. It contains such remarks as 'the government has an interest in the production, distribution, and consumption of alcohol'. These are true statements but very unpalatable to any government.

Another more theoretical example lies in the field of health education. We hear often the message that we must educate the public to lead healthy lives. But the message is not the whole picture. We may advise people to take exercise, to eat brown bread and bran and so on. But we ignore such factors as the higher price of brown bread and its lower availability, or the exercising difficulties of, for example, a single parent in a high rise block. We educate for healthier lifestyles but do not facilitate these. And government, with its complex roles and concern with taxation, distribution, importation and so on, quite often resists this particular role.

The point was also made that there are drawbacks in overstating the role of government as either the source, the tool, or the end-point of implementing preventive health measures. There is a great deal to be said for allowing the value of particular measures to be grasped by the population over time before laws are imposed by the state. Greater reliance on the public conscience or public opinion may lend greater acceptance to an eventual law.

The treatment given to the issue of coercive measures that can be taken by the state has been perhaps too simple and too hostile to the whole concept of coercion. There are a number of instances where coercive measures are a very efficient, simple, and even elegant way of solving problems. If we take the major problem and epidemic of road accidents, some very straighforward coercive measures can help. The facts that within one country it is compulsory to drive on the right hand side of the road or to stop at red traffic lights do impose a certain limitation on personal freedom, but nobody seriously questions those measures. This can be linked to the seat belt question. The French-speaking Swiss were very much opposed to the compulsory use of seat belts when this measure was introduced and remain so, as are the population of the western states of the United States. However, the limitation of freedom in that case is minimal compared with the gains.

An example of limitation of personal freedom where coercive measures would not be justified would be in the prohibition of dangerous activities such as mountain climbing or hang gliding. These are undoubtedly dangerous activities and a number of deaths and accidents are involved. However, the amount of personal pleasure and happiness derived from these activities would make it unacceptable and indeed impossible to prohibit them.

We should beware, therefore, of an over-simplistic treatment of the coercive role of government – there are some simple, elegant, workable coercive measures, and there are others which are unacceptable.

On the different legislative roles of government, it is crucial to distinguish between legislation to promote the health of third parties, such as driving regulations, which tends to be accepted fairly readily, and legislation to promote the health of the individual which is much less easy to justify.

There is, however, a related kind of legislation that is justified and that is legislation to distribute costs fairly. The single most plausible piece of legislation in this context would require separate insurance pools for voluntary risk takers – that is, there should be a requirement on insurance companies to assess risk takers and non risk takers separately in cases where voluntary risks, such as smoking, are involved. This is not an effort to promote health but to distribute costs fairly and it seems a legitimate activity in order to be fair to all in society.

The point was also made in relation to ethical aspects of public health legislation that certain groups, such as those in the army or prisoners, are compelled to take personal risks on occasions in, for example, survival trials or trials of drugs or vaccination. What should the role of medical personnel be in such circumstances?

On the second main theme of discussion – the right to health or to the pursuit of health – more careful examination of the issues was called for. If health is regarded as some final state, in terms of the World Health Organisation definition, then it makes political nonsense to define this as a right or to assign it as an obligation to the state. On the other hand, there is great danger in diluting this to the right to the pursuit of health. Clearly such a statement must be qualified by some assurance that the state will intervene in appropriate instances to ensure a minimum level of wellbeing of all citizens, irrespective of their situation.

One of the dangers of allowing the right to the pursuit of health is that this seems to imply that we are all equal runners in a race. Thus, if we happen to come last in the health race, it is simply bad luck. In fact, as we all know, we are not all equal runners and we must try to even out the inequalities. This must include those inequalities for which we can be held responsible. It is ethically quite unacceptable to attempt to punish people for socially irresponsible behaviour. What happens if someone cannot pay the full cost of the head injury sustained by not wearing a helmet? Is he or she to be allowed to die? The answer here has to be no. If these things happen, people have the right to intervention, at certain minimum levels, whether they can be held responsible or not. The state then has responsibility for legislating in such a way that some of these more irresponsible types of behaviour are prevented. We need a careful examination of both these phrases – right to health and right to pursuit of health. Somewhere in the middle, there are rights to a certain level of human wellbeing which the state has a responsibility to ensure.

For many centuries, discussion on this began not with the right to health but with the duty to preserve yourself in a state of health – a duty to God, society, and yourself. That duty was to be implemented by abstaining from harmful activity and by seeking appropriate medical aid. The duty of the doctor was to help you to preserve your health. The language has changed from duty to right and we are locked into a controversy.

Three other points were raised briefly. The first was that discussion of health economics is difficult because it invokes a type of nonsense discussion. In any society where there is unemployment, human life has a negative value and in such a situation the only cost-effective medical intervention would be abortion.

The second point concerned the complex idea of paying the economic cost of illness. There is a curious paradox with cigarette smoking, for example. There is no doubt that cigarette smoking causes illness and death but it also saves us around £5 billion a year in pensions. It is a question of cost to whom? In this case, if it is cost to the health service, there is a deficit; if it is cost to society as a whole, there is a saving. On the same sort of model, there are those working in the field of liver and kidney transplants who would regret the absence of road traffic accidents.

Finally, in regard specifically to the Oregon experiment, it would be of interest to know the impact of the effort on law-makers, state legislators, senators, congressmen and others, and how a similar approach might be applied in European countries with their very different values, cultures, traditions, and political systems.

CONCLUDING REMARKS

DR PINET

The discussion has been extremely helpful in suggesting possible omissions and some points which I will try to clarify or expand. I have not dealt fully enough perhaps with the conflicts of politics and the potential conflicts between health policies.

I agree also that we cannot equate state and ethics. As we have seen this morning, democratic decisions are taken on the majority principle and it is, therefore, particularly important to recognise the rights of the minority. This is the only way to ensure a democracy. There are of course different types of government or state intervention, alternatives to legislation. Some simple restrictions on freedom have been accepted and are very effective in the public health field.

The role of the third party in any legislative intervention is a very important issue because it introduces an extra and very valid dimension in ethics. In answer to a specific question, I would like to mention here the adoption by the General Assembly of the United Nations in 1983 of the resolution on the 'Principles of medical ethics relevant to the role of health personnel, particularly physicians in the protection of prisoners and detainees against torture and other cruel, inhuman, or degrading treatments or punishment.' I would also like to refer to the 'Proposed international guidelines for biomedical research involving human subjects', elaborated by CIOMS and WHO in 1982.

With regard to the right to health and the right to the pursuit of health, in WHO we have made a study on trends in health legislation in Europe in which the first chapter was devoted to this issue. And it may be appropriate here to remind you of the WHO definition which was mentioned in the discussion : 'the enjoyment of the highest attainable standard of health is one of the fundamental rights of every human being without distinction of race, religion, political belief, economic or social condition'. This definition is often referred to but many people fail to examine carefully the precise terms it uses – it is the highest attainable standard of health, not some absolute right to health. In health law there are two main pillars, the right to self-determination and the right to health care.

The idea of duties rather than rights, I can never accept. Montesquieu wrote that every man who has power tends to abuse his position. The original role of the law was to protect the poor and the less able members of society, and for this we need rights as well as duties.

DR CRAWSHAW

The right to the pursuit of health does not in fact imply that special groups, such as children and old people, should be left out because they cannot compete on equal terms. This right is to protect us from the person who smokes and requires treatment as a consequence and continues to smoke.

I do not think that the Oregon Health Decisions project would have been possible if it had been in any way related to the state. The response of political leaders was mixed. The Governor did not reappoint me to the Health Council, I am without any authority as far as that is concerned. Informally, a number of politicians have come to me for discussion and advice which can be used without acknowledgment. One of the things that we do hope to institute is specific funds for bioethical consultation so that the politicians in the state legislature will have some way of bringing in other kinds of information.

So far as possible European applications of this kind of work are concerned, I am at a loss, but I am fascinated and encouraged by the question. The Club of Rome is the kind of model which might be used since it is independent of government. Governments are not moral or immoral; they are in fact amoral. The only morality we will find for bioethics lies in the population, in people, and it is here that any such experiment must have its base.

ETHICAL ASPECTS OF THE ECONOMICS OF PREVENTION

MARTINE BUNGENER

LEGOS, CNRS, UNIVERSITE DE PARIS IX-DAUPHINE, PARIS

PROFESSOR HARLEM (CHAIRMAN)

I feel very privileged and honoured to be here today, coming out of the cold north to this warm city and to be in such distinguished company. The first paper of Session IV is by Martine Bungener from the Laboratoire d'Economie et de Gestion des Organisations de Santé at the University of Paris IX-Dauphine. It will be presented on her behalf by Dr Blaney.

DR BLANEY FOR DR BUNGENER

This paper concerns the economics of prevention and consists of four parts. First, I would like to discuss the continuing enquiry into the medical effectiveness of prevention and its economic and financial aspects.

Is the enquiry into the economic legitimacy of prevention of the same order as that concerning the cost of illness? Up until the present time, we have tended to concern ourselves more with the economic effectiveness of prevention than with that of medical care. Does this difference arise from the attitude of the medical profession, or from the relationship of the individual human being to questions of health and lifestyle?

The question of the economic effectiveness of prevention depends to a great extent on parallel questions concerning its medical effectiveness. If little information is available about the latter, economic criteria tend to take first place, as we can see when we compare the measures taken to combat cigarette smoking with those concerning perinatal prevention.

This kind of interrogation may be conducted in a number of different ways, including brushing it aside. But by claiming that the object of prevention must not be to reduce health expenditures, or that it has never been proved that prevention has resulted in reducing them, one also implies a concern about its economic effectiveness.

Secondly comes the attempt to evaluate the economic effectiveness of prevention and this illustrates how difficulties arise in terms of appraising and costing the results. These difficulties are amply demonstrated in the diversity of terms used. In French we come across the concepts of 'efficacité' – roughly, effectiveness – and 'advantage', which are used as a basis for so-called 'cost-effectiveness' methods (which compare the results obtained with the means employed without necessarily costing them), and 'cost-advantage' methods (in which results are costed according to a variety of qualitative, quantitative and financial criteria). The English language possesses three specific terms for use in this debate – efficacy, effectiveness, efficiency – which allow a more subtle appraisal of a very complex reality.

The first difficulty is describing the ideal reference situation and we must ask whether this should be economic, medical, or socio-political. The cost argument alone is not sufficient. The fact that calculations point to a certain level of profitability, does not mean that implementing the action will lead to the desired results. Various social or political aspects play a part as does the potential receptivity of the population.

What is the aim of preventive action? Is it to obtain a financial advantage, to improve health status, or a combination of the two? By increasing health status, are we trying to improve individual comfort, or are we seeking increased productivity for society?

The second difficulty relates to evaluating needs. Here we encounter the same difficulties as when we attempt to justify any intervention in the field of health. And these difficulties are increased still further by the difficulty in drawing the line between medical and social needs, because of our recognition of social factors of lifestyle as factors of risk.

The third difficulty relates to evaluating human suffering alleviated and expressing the cost of human lives saved or prolonged. Which components then should we choose? Should we choose leisure, domestic activity, or productivity gains? And how can we integrate these very disparate components. We have to strive for evaluation in monetary terms and taking time lags into account.

The fourth difficulty concerns individual versus community effectiveness. A preventive action which is effective on the individual level may not necessarily be so from the point of view of the community. There is no immediate relationship between microeconomic methods and macroeconomic results. In addition, depending on the type of prevention, the cost may be expressed in terms of individual investment (combatting cigarette smoking) or community consumption (vaccination). This does not allow any immediate comparison between different priority actions nor even with anticipated results.

The micro-macro debate is aggravated by the fact that economic effectiveness must be evaluated within a framework of inelastic global expenditures allocated to medical activity as a whole, both preventive and curative. This raises the specific question of prevention of rare diseases and the apparently inverse question of individual iatrogenic accidents, also very rare, caused by compulsory community prevention.

The fifth difficulty relates to time scale – long-term versus short-term. The economic effectiveness of prevention tends to be presented as an immediate expense which will obviate the need for later expenditures. Apart from the economic problem inherent in any investment choice, corresponding to use of a suitable rate of actualisation, preventive health investment encounters another difficulty related to the financial effectiveness of health expenditures strictly speaking; they may be used to keep alive individuals who later fall sick again and consume medical care which an earlier death would have rendered unnecessary.

Next comes the economic paradox of prevention. Prevention has the effect of diagnosing disease and thus allocating medical expenditure to cure diseases which have remained hitherto undetected and which would otherwise have remained untreated. It can thus result in increased expenditure.

Moreover, if the individual comes to a proper understanding of prevention he will take more interest in his own health and will become more familiar with and more dependent on the health care system. This in turn leads to increased medicalisation and increasing health care expenditure. Thus, paradoxically, prevention leads to increased health expenditure, at least in a preliminary period.

Finally, mention should be made of the ethics and economy of prevention. The ethical aspect of economic questions centres around the decision-making process. The basic question concerns the legitimacy of basing medical decisions on an economic rationale and economic criteria, and the place which should be accorded to these aspects. What importance must we give to the different economic factors in medical decision-making?

Economic logic militates against construction in developing countries of large, technically-equipped hospital complexes which then drain off almost all the country's health resources, despite the fact that such centres would allow individual medical successes. Such logic might also call into question the allocation of funds for expensive therapeutic treatment for an elderly person whose expected lifespan is relatively short. In both cases, the economic argument prefers a collective community choice to the detriment of individual choices, which do not have the same value from an ethical point of view.

The end purpose of medicine is obviously not identical to that of economics. And in both fields, individual objectives may be in conflict with community objectives in a situation where limited resources and cost factors come into play.

Morally speaking we cannot let scarcity of funds engender an unreasoning logic of resource allocation in the health sector, since this would compromise the effectiveness of the whole system of medical care. We must not, however, forget that allocation choices have been made from the beginning, at least implicitly, if not explicitly. It is essential in all circumstances to make them explicit, even if this is painful in a situation of economic crisis. But even if economic aspects have become more important because of the scarcity of funds available, they must never be the only factors to be taken into account. For economics can never be an aim in itself, but must remain solely a means of intervention for attaining objectives agreed upon by the community.

DISCUSSION

Discussants: Harlem (Chairman), Beauchamp, Pochin, Tognoni

Three main points were raised on Dr Bungener's paper.

The first was in relation to long and short-term effects, where there is an agent – for example, ionising radiation – which will cause effects at a later date, either in future generations or in terms of long-life radioactive materials. A biologist would attach the same importance to a death or a genetic defect occurring in 50 or 100 years as to a similar defect occurring in the present generation. An economist, asked to make provision for these kinds of harm, however, would apply a form of discounting which would attach zero importance to death at many years in the future. This is a real dilemma when one is considering the importance of these late effects, either biologically or in terms of national provision of health care.

Secondly, it was felt that this paper should include some comments on how economics actually deals with medicine. Attention is usually focussed on the conflicting demands for health expenditure and the economic reality of limited resources. But how in fact do we face up to this conflict and try to resolve the dilemma? How does it work in practice?

The third point concerned a problem that is considered very important in the United States and also perhaps in Europe – that is the way in which cost-benefit is raised to the level of a high political principle. According to this philosophy, we will not intervene in any area, including health, unless the benefits are so great that they outweigh considerations of economic cost. The argument is made that we should only intervene, whether we are regulating in the case of transport or of health, in a manner that produces a net gain in economic efficiency.

At least in the United States, that has never been a principle at law. In fact in the development of the constitutional tradition in the United States, when one, for example, employed regulatory or police power to regulate a piece of property, it was never required that we compensated the person whose property we regulated in order to redress the loss of value of their property to protect the public health. It was always recognised that the value of the public health was higher in priority than was economic value. If, on the other hand, we took over someone's land to build a public road, they were entitled to compensation. This is more like the principle of cost-benefit and in fact the Kaldor-Hicks equation is built precisely on this principle of compensation.

Perhaps this whole notion of cost-benefit as a limiting political principle is one that needs to be discussed. It is in some ways far more dangerous than the whole argument about how much a human life is worth, contentious though that is. Surely we cannot substitute economic principles for political principles and a democratic people must resist vigorously the idea that they should only intervene and use the government's power when it is economically beneficial to do so.

CONCLUDING REMARKS

DR BUNGENER

On the first point, it is of course true that there is in economics a discounting rate that does not apply in medicine, ethics, or biology in all of which contexts one death equals one death. But it is also a general principle in economics that the discount rate can be adjusted according to the logic of the situation.

On the second point, there have been several recent examples where economics were not not a very good instrument of prevision. However, economics remains a useful instrument of analysis, of explanation, and of understanding reality, even if it is imperfect, and it is certainly of value in the health field.

On the third point, economics and notions of cost-benefit should clearly be subsumed under health policy, not the reverse.

ETHICAL ISSUES IN DESCRIPTIVE AND ANALYTICAL EPIDEMIOLOGY AND IN PRIMARY PREVENTION

E G KNOX

HEALTH SERVICES RESEARCH CENTRE, DEPARTMENT OF SOCIAL MEDICINE, UNIVERSITY OF BIRMINGHAM, BIRMINGHAM

PROFESSOR HARLEM (CHAIRMAN)

I now have pleasure in introducing the next speaker, Professor George Knox, who is Head of the Department of Social Medicine at Birmingham University.

PROFESSOR KNOX

Before addressing my main theme, I should say that two separate classes of ethical problem arise out of epidemiological research. The first relates to its field of application and the second to the methods which it uses. In relation to its field of application, epidemiological research can of course be used for many other purposes than health. It is used for advertising, selling toothpaste, selling drugs, biological warfare, agriculture – a large range of applications. In these non-health applications, special ethical problems arise from the applications themselves, particularly if they use human data which were collected from patients under the pretext of another objective. For the remainder of my presentation I would like to concentrate specifically on applications of epidemiology to health and health care problems where this kind of issue does not arise.

Epidemiology within that context traditionally relates to prevention but not purely so. Nowadays it is concerned also with the evaluation of health care services, including therapeutic services and caring services. Community Medicine, or Social Medicine, or Public Health, now has a fairly comprehensive responsibility for all divisions of health care services. Within this broad field the three objectives quoted by Dr Bungener – efficacy, effectiveness and efficiency – are the main targets towards which epidemiological research is directed. This is especially true of the efficacy of procedures and the effectiveness of programmes; efficiency is usually regarded as a more purely administrative objective.

I would also like to comment on the psychology of the way in which many people understand research. Those that do the research believe, as I do, that the dependence of medicine upon research is total – that is, we do not find out anything except by research, research is our only source of knowledge. Most people here would accept that. I mention it only because there are many who do not think like that at all. They think of research as a kind of optional academic extra. It is necessary therefore to assert that research is an absolute necessity, that lives depend on it, and that we get nowhere without it.

Sometimes we hear complaints that we are asking people to take risks or suffer inconvenience for the sake of research. Let us therefore declare again that research has not got a 'sake'. People are being asked to contribute for the benefit of other people. One person is being asked to take a risk, to suffer inconvenience, or to sacrifice something, for the benefit of somebody else; not for the benefit of the research.

I was asked to consider descriptive and analytical types of research but it is difficult to separate them. Very seldom do we do just one and not the other. Descriptive research asks 'where did it happen; when did it happen; who did it happen to; what is the incidence or prevalence; and how is it distributed in the population?' Analytical research is simply the next stage. We go on to make inferences about causes and about aetiology. By this we mean the causes which precede the onset of the disease. Pathologists often speak of cause in a different way. They are concerned with the ways in which one pathological feature of a disease leads to another, and then causes its symptoms and signs. They are concerned with the internal mechanisms of the disease; the mechanisms they hope can be interrupted. Naturally enough, people concerned with cure and with therapy are interested in causes in this particular sense. It is usually called 'pathogenesis'.

Those involved in prevention are, however, concerned especially with the causes which precede the disease; that is, its aetiology. And although epidemiology is sometimes referred to as an abstract science, it is in this kind of application very specifically related to devising preventive mechanisms.

Both descriptive and analytical work are essentially passive in that they are based on observation and not upon manipulation or intervention. In one of the other papers, there is some description of the uses of randomised trials. That, of course, is intervention and introduces additional ethical problems. However, the kind of work I am speaking about is pure observation. It is descriptive and analytical. The main ethical problems are infringements of privacy or of confidentiality.

I have been Chairman of a Working Group of the EEC which has been looking into this and trying to reconcile the right to privacy on the one hand and the duty to contribute to research for the benefit of fellow members of society on the other. Many of my subsequent remarks spring from this experience.

The traditional approach is that of Hippocrates, declaring strict medical secrecy. Nowadays this is 'modified' so that there are many people besides the doctor who are allowed to look at medical records. What we are saying really is that strict medical secrecy is, in many cases, rather a myth. Medical information is not widely spread; but it is not very closely controlled either. There are two dangers. One is that confidentiality becomes so disregarded that no one can trust their doctor any more. The other is that doctors become so defensive that epidemiological research becomes totally impossible.

This is where the main ethical problem of practical epidemiology now lies. As someone has already said, it is not a conflict between good and bad; it is a conflict between two principles of equal merit. These are the most important and the most subtle of the ethical problems which we face. If it were a straight choice between good and bad, or between what we consider to be good and bad, it would be fairly easy. But a conflict between principles of equal merit raises real difficulties.

How can we attempt to solve the dilemma? Our working group first took some legal advice: and the legal advice was not to take legal advice! Lawyers, on the whole, tend to operate through sets of rules and there was no set of rules here which could reconcile the conflict without compromising one or other objective. We should note that this is not a conflict arising from extrinsic circumstances which could be altered, like a shortage of resources; and it is not a conflict born of stupidity or obtuseness on our part. It is a problem which really has no answer at all. It is an insoluble, indelible, absolute, and forever kind of conflict and there is nothing that we can do to make it go away.

Faced with a problem of this sort, what kind of advice can we give? Is it perhaps an issue outside the area of ethics altogether, and simply a question of power, and perhaps of majority and minority views?

Although these issues were highlighted in relation to confidentiality, I have met this kind of problem in other contexts. I have been Chairman of a Committee on Fluoridation in the United Kingdom, looking specifically at the issue of an alleged connection between cancer and fluoride. There is very good evidence that the supposed connection is totally spurious, but we are left with a conflict. Some people wish to have fluoride in their water supply, and some people do not. To one group, fluoride is a beneficial public health measure which is being obstructed by others; to another group, it is 'mass medication' being enforced by others. Even if the scientific issues of benefit and safety have been resolved and a majority consensus reached, the issue remains as to whether those who do not wish to have fluoride in their water, should be compelled to take fluoride because the majority wish it.

Vaccination raises another major ethical conflict. In measles vaccination, when you vaccinate people, you do them good. You also do good to the people whom you did not vaccinate because you protect them against the rapid spread of measles and you postpone the measles (if they get it at all) to an age where they more easily withstand the illness and suffer less harm.

In the case of rubella, you also do good to those to whom you give the vaccine, or rather to their children when they grow up. But you do harm to those to whom you do not give the vaccine. It works like this. If you give vaccine to half the population, that half is protected. However, the disease in the other half is delayed and this is serious in the case of rubella because infection in adult age groups puts children at risk from Congenital Rubella Syndrome (CRS).

Depending on the mode of transmission in a particular population, the net effect can be that, with a vaccine uptake rate of about 50%, you might cause as many cases of CRS as you prevent. All you achieve is to redistribute the disease to different people. Net benefit depends on uptake rates of more than 50% but some people are still being harmed. Only if uptake rises to around 95% or more can you get total benefit and not cause harm. And to achieve this, vaccination must usually be made compulsory – except in Sweden where they have such methods of persuasion that they can do it without compulsion!

This presents a very difficult policy choice. Here is a disease which we wish to eradicate by vaccination. But for this to be effective and not to cause harm, the vaccination would have to be made compulsory. We have a conflict. It is usually described as a conflict between the individual and society, but society is composed of people, and it is really a conflict between some people and other people. This is the worst kind of conflict; the one that will not go away.

To summarise, we identified a species of problem, exemplified in the areas of confidentiality of records, fluoridation, and rubella vaccination, which are essentially insoluble. There is no formal answer or solution to them. They are not susceptible to universal formal rules. We must find some other way of handling them.

The solution adopted by the EEC Working Party on Confidentiality, and incidentally by other national bodies looking at the same problem, was to devise a Code of

Practice, without force of law but to which reference could be made within legal provisions. There are analogies in the United Kingdom with the Highway Code – the code of driving practice. In some respects this represents a retreat from ethics and from the law. Certainly it is not a solution, but rather a pragmatic response to a situation which has no solution. It has disadvantages in that it invokes judgment regarding a balance of interests and regarding the needs of individuals and of communities. This in turn presents difficulties in that the assessment of need is always a concept in the mind of the provider. In its adoption we are forced back into the adoption of a paternalistic mode of thought; and then we must ask whose paternalism? Public bodies; doctors; legislators; professional organisations? In our EEC report we opted for doctors. We can be accused of being prejudiced. For the moment, however, we see no real alternative.

DISCUSSION

Discussants: Harlem (Chairman), Blaney, Canosa, Dunstan, Gorovitz, Martin, Nicholson, Pochin, Riis, Sand, Terborgh-Dupuis, Veatch, Zakopoulos, Zander

Discussion on Professor Knox's paper began with some comments on the distinction between clinical and epiedmiological research. Discussion then centred on the question of conflicts of interests, particularly in relation to the the issues of confidentiality versus the need for research and compulsion versus respect for individual liberty.

The distinction between clinical research and epidemiological research was stressed again. Clinical research deals with ill people, people with some kind of medical condition which requires attention. In this situation people are very vulnerable to research. They tend to agree very willingly to research procedures because they feel that refusal may hinder their recovery and prejudice their doctor's attitude to them. Epidemiological research in contrast deals with healthy people who are not in hospital beds and so who are not actually dependent on the paternal role of the doctor for their future and advice. As anybody who has carried out epidemiological research knows well, we are dealing with the free animal out in the wild, who needs to be hunted down, as it were, needs to be cajoled, persuaded – an entirely different approach. Unfortunately, when it comes to questions of consent or confidentiality, the principles or codes that we have applied to individual currently sick patients in clinical research tend to be applied to epidemiological research. We have to beware also of over-ambitious, competitive researchers – what people often fear is not running risks for the sake of science but for the sake of scientists. There must be some protection here.

There are major ethical problems in the use of epidemiological data – that is, the outcome of research. Most research results are difficult to interpret beause of their multivariate character. The 'causal' factors usually explain only a small part of the condition which is supposed to be 'prevented'. The question is: how can we define or discuss the proportion of causality which is a limit leading to preventive intervention?

Another problem that arises in epidemiological research is that of control groups. In long-term epidemiological studies, such as those on smoking, nutritional supplements, cardiovascular disease, low birth weight and so on, control groups are vital. And we need to address ourselves to the ethical implications of involving perfectly healthy individuals in long-term research. An example was given from a study in Guatemala involving two groups of pregnant women – one group was given food supplements and the other was not. However, both groups received medical care and regular supervision and that fact in itself changed the nature of the control group. The experiment itself, the very fact of being in a control group with increased attention and increased awareness, is going to change the group.

In purely descriptive epidemiological research, many people would say that if anonymous data are involved there are no ethical problems. But even here the problem of stigmatisation can arise in selected groups even where individuals cannot be identified. One project that was quoted in illustration of this involved young girls who had been victims of incest – any follow-up to assess possible damage they may have suffered, might stigmatise them in a very harmful way.

If we move to community or preventive research involving intervention, a project was described in which a large group of old people was randomised to one group that had home visits from doctors and nurses and a control group which did not receive such visits. After several years, it became evident that those being visited at home had fewer visits to hospital and lower mortality than the control group. In this case, there was no intervention at all in the private lives of the control group and the ethical balance was perhaps more simple.

In the example of vaccination, most programmes have been carried out without control groups and there are thus many results that cannot be properly interpreted. To do such research properly, there must be control groups, and the ethical balance is difficult.

The issue of conflicting interests is a central one in any ethical discussions and the approach of representative democracy is perhaps the best available system. There are three main ways in which those in the fields of medicine and ethics can qualify political decisions in this area – by education, by analysis, and by debate.

Confidentiality is a critical issue in epidemiological research, and one that involves a central conflict of interests. It is one of the dilemmas described by Professor Knox as insoluble. In the United States at least, however, there have been no fewer than three solutions regarding the use of records for epidemiological research.

One technical fix is simply to attach an explicit consent to medical records waiving confidentiality for epidemiological research. Thus individuals waive their claim of confidentiality and it is universally recognised that a right of confidentiality can be waived by the holder of that right.

Secondly, and this is a little more complicated, it is possible to construct a consent for the use of the record. This is done in American legal form, by asking what would a reasonable person want to know before his record is used? If the answer to that question is 'nothing' – that is to say he would not want to be told about it – one has in effect constructed a consent for the use of the record for this purpose. It would require testing to see whether the record contains any potentially controversial information or whether there is controversy in the purpose of the research. Finally, one might override the confidentiality claim of the individual by appealing to the principle of justice, not simply to the principle of the aggregate benefit to be gained. A combination of these three maneouvres should normally be adequate to justify any reasonable record search.

The practical point was made that there are some countries or districts within countries in which death certificates, recording the cause of death of individuals, are understandably confidential documents. However, in some countries the death certificate can be torn in half – the lower half records the cause of death and the means of identifying the cause, unrelated to the name of the individual. This allows fields for epidemiological research which are important without a real breach of confidentiality, provided there is a mechanism at the registration of causes of death which will link the cause of death with the individual without disclosing this.

A striking contrast has arisen between those like Professor Knox who view the intractable conflict between the two principles of respect for confidentiality and the need for epidemiological research as an insoluble dilemma and those who respond to this by suggesting three immediate ways to resolve it.

In a sense both viewpoints are justified as an examination of the methodology of attempts to resolve the conflict can show. The description of the situation as one in which there is no solution is uncomfortable because the moral problem is, given that conflict of principles, what do we do and why, how do we act? That is always a solvable problem, even when we face that problem in the context of a clash of principles, neither of which will give way to the other.

What is the range of options open to the person facing that conflict of principles? One is to abandon the epidemiological research. Another is to disregard the concern for confidentiality. Both of those are unacceptable. In fact the response that was described was one which seeks to minimise the moral damage by charting a course of action that pays maximum respect to the two principles. Knowing that it does not respect either of them perfectly, or completely, it is a course of action that violates to the minimum extent the combination of these two principles. There is a sense in which a recipient of medical care is the beneficiary of a public good, the possibility of medical treatment. There is a reasonable argument that some conditions of reciprocity apply, that one owes in response some cooperation, some partial diminution of absolute privacy. At the same time, the researchers have a responsibility to conduct the research in a way that violates that confidentiality to the minimum possible degree.

There are then some action imperatives that follow from this sort of situation. These are, on the one hand, to remove the identifiers in the way that was described, to maintain records carefully and conscientiously, and to control access. And on the other hand, there must be open and assertive encouragement of the notion that there is a responsibility on recipients of medical care to participate at minimum or low risk in activities that carry medical research forward generally. Thus the ethical approach is not to try to dissolve the conflict of principles but to try to determine a mode of action within the context of the conflict that minimises the extent to which we violate the principles.

The other main conflict of interests which arose in discussion was that illustrated in the rubella example, the conflict of compulsion versus individual freedom, and many of the arguments described above can also be applied to this. The rubella example is a very special case where it was suggested a straightforward policy of compulsory immunisation of the female population at least can easily be justified on grounds of direct and obvious benefits to third parties – that is, future offspring. It is a very special case in the immunisation debate. It may be in this particular instance, that compulsory vaccination is justified. People can claim two kinds of rights – rights to freedom or liberty and rights that make it necessary for others to provide some commodity or service. But, if people want something, then they must be prepared to give something. If they want to be healthy, they have to give up some rights of liberty and we should not persist in regarding this as a problem.

On the other hand, anxiety was expressed on the statement that the only way to get a 95 per cent uptake of immunisation is by legislation. In the case of rubella, there are examples of schools in England where the clinical medical officers responsible for providing rubella immunisation for schoolgirls have made a real effort to educate the girls about the disease and about congenital rubella syndrome in infants, and uptake rates have risen to over 90 per cent without any form of compulsion. It is too simplistic to say that there must be legislation for a particular form of prevention when there are ways of achieving this which also protect people's freedom to make choices.

This dilemma between individual freedom of choice and what is best for the community as a whole is central to our whole subject. One element which we should consider is the dynamic one of change of attitude. We have tended to think of the question of individual liberty as something which remains unchanged and which must be protected at all costs. The seat belt discussion in Britain is a case in point. This discussion was exceedingly vociferous and went on for a long time. The issue of individual rights was strong and central until the law had been passed. Since then there has been almost no discussion at all and the results have been seen to be beneficial. So we have to try to introduce a dynamic dimension into individual rights, to be prepared to take a decision and then amend or enforce it as circumstances demand. We cannot accept these conflicts and dilemmas as insoluble. We have to provide solutions.

CONCLUDING REMARKS

PROFESSOR KNOX

On the differences between clinical and epidemiological research, it is quite true that in preventive medicine the research subjects can be in good or reasonable health, and we should bear in mind the differences from clinical research. However, epidemiological research also on occasion involves people who are sick, particularly in the case-control approach. The example of neural tube defects illustrates this nicely. This condition is much more common in Britain than in the rest of Europe and has a social, geographical, and seasonal distribution which strongly suggests an environmental, probably dietary, causation. In the past it has been impossible to carry out a satisfactory case-control study to explore this, since women cannot usually remember their precise diet during pregnancy, eight or nine months later. With the advent of early abortion following screening tests, the memory time-lag is much shorter, and there is some hope of conducting an effective case-control comparison. However, if we dive into that delicate situation between the obstetrician and his patient, it becomes very difficult. First there is a test because something might be wrong; then there is another test because something is wrong; and after exploration and discussion an abortion is offered. Any research intervention in the middle of all that raises very serious practical and ethical difficulties.

The problem of fear of scientists rather than of science was raised. This anti-expert, anti-authority feeling is real, and a serious pragmatic obstruction; but it is not a moral or ethical problem. The feeling is currently so strong in some countries that it is almost impossible even to carry out a census.

On the rubella question I should have said that there are two possible policies. One is to vaccinate schoolgirls. We call this the indirect method, because it does not eliminate rubella, but provides protection from the consequences of exposure. By age 20, 22, or 25 years, the majority of subjects are immune because of natural exposure, not because of the vaccine; the vaccine acts as a supplement. The alternative policy is to vaccinate both boys and girls at the age of 1 to 2 years in combination with mumps and measles vaccines. If that policy is undertaken successfully, the disease is eliminated. The result is therefore more satisfactory, although vaccination must be maintained to prevent reintroduction. However, if the implementation falls short, and the disease is not eradicated, there is a terrible risk of a huge epidemic, later. This is an unacceptable risk to take on behalf of a population unless there is a guarantee of a long continuing high level of uptake of vaccination. My judgment, and the judgment of many others, is that the risk is so severe that this particular policy should not be adopted unless vaccination is made compulsory. The real dilemma is not whether to vaccinate at all, but whether to go for eradication of rubella or control of CRS. The latter policy is much more sluggish in its response and many lives are lost in the 20 years it takes to have effect. An eradication policy successfully applied, as in the United States, takes only 10 years to show its main benefits. But if it falls short, then the loss of life is greater still.

The central point of our discussion, however, was the question of insoluble conflicts between, for example, confidentiality and the need for research, and between compulsion for the common good and self-determination. There is an intellectual repugnance, which I share, to the notion of there being no solutions to certain kinds of problems. Scientists feel this most of all because the primary scientific premise is that the world is consistent and a conflict which has no solution disturbs this basic idea. (We are speaking of situations with no solutions, rather than solutions which we are unable to find.) This is probably the case also with lawyers. They are happy enough with conflict. That is the main material of their lives. But they work on the principle that there are rules to deal with it. Politicians, on the other hand, take conflict for granted. And irreconcilable conflict, at that. The whole essence of politics is conflict, and conflicts that are settled by power processes, or by negotiation if not imposition, and not by logical resolution. There are two worlds here. All is well so long as we keep the lawyers, the politicians, and the scientists apart, but difficulties arise whenever these two worlds meet and we have to bridge the gap between them.

When there are two incompatible principles of merit, there is no solution in the sense of making them compatible. The best we can do is to seek a way to minimise the physical, moral, and ethical damage, as was so elegantly stated in the discussion.

ETHICAL ISSUES IN TRIALS OF PREVENTION

T STRASSER

DEPARTMENT OF SOCIAL AND PREVENTIVE MEDICINE, UNIVERSITY OF GENEVA, GENEVA

DR D ROY (CHAIRMAN)

I would like to open this morning's session with a brief quotation on one aspect of prevention quite different from the one that we will be concentrating on this morning. It comes from an article by W Hutchinson in the Journal of the American Medical Association: 'The system of remuneration makes the physicians's income dependent on the amount of sickness. Our system's philosophy might be condensed in the motto, millions for care and not one cent for prevention. It seems to me the weakness of our system lies in this one fact that it gives physicians such exceedingly limited opportunity for what has been called the practice of preventive medicine'. This was published on 30 October 1886, almost 100 years ago. Whether or not we are today beginning to give millions for prevention, prevention trials are the subject of our next speaker, Dr Toma Strasser. Dr Strasser is Visiting Professor at the Department of Social and Preventive Medicine, University of Geneva, and Professor of Medicine at the University of Novi Sad in Yugoslavia. He has been Secretary General of the World Hypertension League and consultant to the World Health Organisation.

DR STRASSER

My co-authors, Dr Jeanneret and Dr Raymond, and myself have a longstanding interest in medical ethics and we have been collaborating for many years on prevention trials in children. In the limited time at my disposal today, however, I would like to deal mainly with two topics particularly relevant to ethical issues in prevention trials in general. I will talk about the complexity of ethical issues, and about the responsibility for interpreting the outcome of trials. If time permits, I shall also mention briefly the questions of informed consent in population or community studies, the relativity of values, and the levels of certitude. In doing this I shall illustrate the points by using the case histories of two particular trials. As a practising epidemiologist I shall not deal with the theoretical aspects which have already been fully and competently discussed.

The complexity of ethical issues is nicely illustrated by the first case history. In the mid 1960s it became clear that the lipid hypothesis of atherogenesis had a solid basis, established by descriptive epidemiological studies. But it remained to be tested whether an intervention on the lowering of serum lipids would prevent coronary heart disease. A primary prevention trial of coronary heart disease was, therefore, set up. Clofibrate was given to a large number of healthy people in a controlled trial, with a control group which was given olive oil as placebo and another control group which was simply observed. The results of the trial showed that long-term administration of clofibrate does lower serum cholesterol and reduces the incidence of non-fatal coronary heart disease by something like 20 per cent. But this beneficial effect of clofibrate was negated by an excess mortality observed in the clofibrate group compared with the group which was receiving olive oil.

I would like now to make a brief *post-festum* analysis of the justification of this study. Was the intervention trial ethically justified or not? It must of course be remembered that at the time when the trial was planned and started, there was much less concern about the ethical aspects of such research. It would be much more difficult to undertake such a study today and, with hindsight, I do not think I would participate in it. Analysis of the justification of the trial produces several positives and several negatives. From the modern viewpoint, the trial was not justified ecologically. Serum lipids can be lowered by natural means and there can, therefore, be no justification for lowering them chemically. When I calculated this morning the total amount of clofibrate given in this trial over the years, it amounted to 30 tons or 30 million grams. Thus if we recognise the ethical importance of the preservation of the chemical or physical environment the trial was not justified. On the other hand, the trial was justified, paradoxically, because of the negative outcome. If the trial had not been carried out, clofibrate would not have been discredited and would have continued to be given over many decades to come in unlimited quantities.

There is another positive in the fact that the study has confirmed the lipid hypothesis of atherogenesis. That was an unplanned 'side-product' of the trial but an important scientific gain. Another negative, on the other hand, lies in the fact that, although the trial demonstrated that clofibrate is inappropriate for primary prevention of ischaemic heart disease, the result has simply been a shift in the prescribing habits of doctors. They started prescribing other drugs from the same family, for example, fenofibrate or bezafibrate, instead. These are not the same as clofibrate but similar and with probably similar effects. And since they have not been tested, they continue to be given. Looked at from this point of view, the trial was not justified because it has not led to a radical change in medical practice. It has merely had a superficial effect on prescribing and this introduces the complex issue of implementation of results and the impact of such a trial on actual medical and behavioural practice.

There are now two negatives and two positives in our justification analysis but there is a third positive. The intervention itself has still done more good than harm, because the excess mortality was only a relative one – that is to say, there was a higher mortality in the clofibrate group than in the placebo control group, but the latter group had an unusually low mortality, far below that of the general population. So the study did good to the placebo group and the excess mortality was purely relative.

This kind of analysis or 'autopsy' highlights the complexity of the ethical issues involved in such a trial. The difficulty, however, lies in how we can possibly foresee all such issues when planning and seeking approval for this kind of research.

The question of responsibility in interpreting research results can be shown in the case history of the very famous multiple risk factor intervention trial which has been called, in our cardiovascular epidemiological jargon, the MRFIT trial. In the mid 1970s it became evident, again on the basis of descriptive studies, that coronary heart disease and atherosclerosis are associated with multiple risk factors. But it remained to be shown that intervention on those risk factors would produce a reduction in the incidence of coronary heart disease. An expensive, complicated, and well-executed trial was carried out on a large number of healthy individuals in order to change their lifestyles and reduce coronary risk. The trial, which ended recently, has produced a very modest result with almost no discernible effect on reducing the incidence of coronary heart disease. While the trial was in progress, further evidence indicated clearly that a lowering of risk factor levels in the population is associated with a fall in coronary mortality in a number of countries, including the United States and Australia. So some more indirect evidence became available on the efficacy of lowering risk factor level.

The interpretation of the results of the multiple risk factor intervention trial, therefore, carries a very great responsibility. Here is a trial which has failed to demonstrate the benefits of multiple risk intervention. Is this an argument against intervening on the risk factors even in the presence of other circumstantial evidence? The issue at stake is a crucial one because it does not involve tens or dozens of individuals but the definition of health policies and recommendations for thousands and hundreds of thousands of people. There is a huge risk and an awesome responsibility in interpreting the failure to demonstrate the effectiveness of preventing a potentially preventable disease as an indication for negative or non-existent advice. The problems of interpretation are thus immense.

There are many other issues which we may touch on in discussion, such as informed consent of a community, the relativity of various values which may influence the interpretation of prevention trials, or the formulation of prevention policies. Should smoking, for example, be advised against vigorously in elderly people, with an obviously reduced life expectancy, who have smoked all their lives and in whom such an intervention might cause more distress than benefit? On the other hand elderly persons should clearly not be deprived of the advances of medicine. These are complicated ethical issues which we must face.

I would like to end by suggesting a kind of credo: to try to influence the health-related values of society should be a standing commitment of the medical profession. This is a typical prescriptive statement with which Ivan Illich I am sure would disagree. I should appreciate some discussion of its validity. It leads naturally to the possibly provocative conclusion that even the best prevention studies are not fully justified unless we can sell the results to health policy-makers and society at large.

DISCUSSION

Discussants: Roy (Chairman), Beauchamp, Blaney, Campbell, Crawshaw, Doxiadis, Gorovitz, Martin, Mumuftu, Pinet, Riis, Sand, Tatsis, Tognoni, Veatch, Violaki, Zakopoulos, Zander

The discussion on Dr Strasser's paper concerned two main aspects – the question of informed consent and the credo mentioned at the end of his presentation.

Informed consent is a condition for performing controlled trials in clinical medicine in the developed countries and it is becoming accepted now that it ought to be a global condition. In the developed countries, populations still have many difficulties in accepting the principle of the two or three groups to which patients are allocated at random. Indeed many journalists and other representatives of the population still refer to the original statement of the first Helsinki declaration as meaning that you are allowed to undertake controlled trials only if you can be sure they will be beneficial to the participants. This is of course nonsense in logical terms since if we knew the answers, we would not be carrying out the trial.

In preventive medicine or health promotion where it may be desirable to test large scale measures under controlled conditions, the situation on informed consent is even more difficult. The example of speed limits is one illustration of some of the problems. Discussions over many years have suggested that a reduction in the speed limit would reduce road traffic accidents, a major cause of mortality and morbidity in most countries. A controlled trial could have been carried out, for example, in perhaps two French provinces compared with the rest of that country, or in northern Denmark, but this was not accepted, and it seems doubtful whether this principle of informed consent by proxy will ever be accepted in the developed countries. There is therefore, a risk which we must guard against of simply exporting this problem to the developing countries and importing the results so that we have elegant clinical trials in one context and large scale preventive trials in another. The policy of WHO and CIOMS in this field is extremely important to ensure that we avoid exporting our ethical problems. We need preventive trials of course and this presupposes informed consent but we have a responsibility to create the results and deal with the problems in our own communities.

Once again the difference between clinical and preventive medicine was stressed. What we require from an individual taking part in a clinical trial is informed consent in the knowledge of any possible side-effects in terms of their health, their wellbeing, or their chances of dying. The necessity for informed consent is thus very important indeed in cases where there is a possible risk to health or life. It is less important when there is no obvious immediate risk.

Over-emphasis on these clinical elements of informed consent, transferred without question from the clinical setting, poses a definite threat to epidemiological research. One of the basic requirements in taking a sample of the general population, with regard, for example, to the prevalence or incidence of a particular condition, is that the sample should be representative of the total population. And if the sample is to be representative, a certain proportion of that sample – 75 to 85 per cent – should cooperate in the study. If we make informed consent in this context too involved and too complicated, this percentage is likely to drop to an unacceptable level. In one study of lead levels in a particular population in Ireland, for example, the research worker clearly misunderstood the implications of the informed consent required. Each individual in the sample was asked to sign their name on a consent form to confirm their willingness to participate. The cooperation rate was 25 per cent. A possible compromise was suggested in using specific groups, such as doctors and nurses, as reference populations in some instances. This has already been done with trials of vitamin A in the United States and aspirin in Britain.

A complication arises in research concerning children. Traditional wisdom recognised the right of the parent or guardian to decide on behalf of the child. But this concept has come under increasing fire in the light of the growing recognition of children's rights and abuses on the part of research, especially in developed countries. The family, however, remains the most fundamental unit in society, and if parents cannot decide for their children, who can? No one questions parents' rights to allow their child to participate in activities involving greater potential risks than most research – riding in a car, for example, or going swimming, horseback riding, skiing, or camping. Parents control all aspects of their young children's lives so why should their right to decide whether or not they should be involved in research be questioned, provided they are well informed on the matter.

A final point on informed consent is that there are instances where information vitiates the point of the research. Paediatricians, for example, are currently anxious to know more about the effects of alcohol and drug abuse in pregnant women on the foetus and the newborn. If this is presented as a research project, the subjects are likely to try to conceal or underplay their use of alcohol or drugs and the investigation will be meaningless.

The second aspect for discussion on Dr Strasser's presentation concerned the wider issue of a credo in preventive and population survey. Can such surveys be an end in themselves or should they produce some benefit to the population involved? The example was given of nutritional surveys in developing countries, or even in some developed countries. If the results of such a trial demonstrated a nutritional deficiency without the option to correct or at least lessen the deficiency, we are faced with the ethics of false hope. This has wide repercussions in terms of the morale of the research workers, the disappointment of the population, and the indifference or false satisfaction of the government.

There is also of course the opposite point of view that if we never undertake research projects without the assurance of a benefit to the population, we are not going to sensitise governments or other responsible agents to unfulfilled health needs. So the question of guaranteed beneficial outcome is complex and has clear ethical implications. If there is benefit, we must also distinguish between the long-term and the short-term. There is a nutritional deficiency of vitamin A which causes an eye disease leading to blindness. A population with this deficiency in children can be investigated and the problem treated with drops of vitamin A to avoid blindness. But with this short-term benefit, there is the danger of overlooking the need to produce a long-term benefit – the general correction of the nutritional deficiency which is much more extensive.

So what should we be looking for in our credo? Is it enough simply to state 'to try to influence the health-related values of society should be a standing commitment of the medical profession?' One element which we have not fully recognised is that the health care professions are not in themselves united. We are talking about the ethical problems of persuading the population of the benefits of our research. But at the end of the clofibrate story, we were told that, after this long study with all its implications, behaviour did not change. Clinicians are now prescribing almost identical substances and their justification for this is that there has been no study on these. So we need research, we need these studies, but are we really sure that our results actually influence medical behaviour at all? What we must work on is this intraprofessional relationship, and the cooperation of clinicians is an essential part of meaningful research. A commitment on the part of other influential groups in society is also essential.

Dr Strasser was complimented on working towards a credo and on providing an example of active ethical intervention and involvement. This is in marked contrast to the passive attitudes so characteristic of much research – namely, have we fulfilled all the official requirements; if so, there is no need to think about ethics at all. However, the use of the phrase 'standing commitment of the medical profession' inclines towards a kind of ivory tower sense of the credo. We should perhaps encourage rather the use of a more positive phrase such as 'interdependent commitment of all involved in health care research', including of course, the patients.

CONCLUDING REMARKS

DR STRASSER

I am most grateful for such a rich discussion. The point on intraprofessional relationships and responsibilities ties up well with the points made for and against the health care professions acting as advocates or evangelists for health. This is not a new issue, it is one which causes much discussion and disagreement within the medical profession, and it does present real theoretical problems.

I would like to close with one reflection. Among the words used several times this morning were coercion and conditioning. Also implied in several of the interventions was the concept of persuasion which is one of the functions of civilised discourse. And it seems to me, as one of the contributors mentioned, that we should move in the direction of a more vivid return to persuasion as one of the instruments of prevention.

ETHICAL ISSUES OF HEALTH PROMOTION, HEALTH EDUCATION, AND BEHAVIOURAL CONTROL

LEON EISENBERG

DEPARTMENT OF SOCIAL MEDICINE AND HEALTH POLICY, HARVARD UNIVERSITY MEDICAL SCHOOL, BOSTON

DR ROY (CHAIRMAN)

The second paper of this session will now be presented by Dr Doxiadis on behalf of Dr Leon Eisenberg who is unfortunately unable to be here. Dr Eisenberg is an eminent child psychiatrist and Professor of Social Medicine and Health Policy at Harvard University Medical School.

DR DOXIADIS FOR DR EISENBERG

I would like to begin by summarising the main points of Dr Eisenberg's paper and will then add some comments of my own. We have then invited Professor Gorovitz to make a short initial comment before the main discussion.

Dr Eisenberg begins by stressing the need for definitions of three terms – health promotion, health education, and behavioural control. Each of these activities occurs inevitably but in an unplanned way in all human societies. What distinguishes them in modern society is that they are planned and that they are based on what is understood by experts and specialists rather than on what is shared knowledge in the community.

Although the importance of randomised controlled trials is widely accepted as a necessary step in evaluating new medications and procedures, health promotion and health education are commonly regarded as having face validity and are usually introduced without systematic evaluation.

Programmes for health promotion through education have differential effects by social class with the higher social classes the most likely to profit from typical educational interventions. Public health programmes must, therefore, take into account the social forces which impede the adoption of 'healthy lifestyles' by disadvantaged segments of the population. Furthermore, programmes to encourage health promoting behaviour must be adapted to the meanings of behaviour in particular cultures and to the values which guide them. All too often, what is considered optimal for middle-class Caucasian men is recommended for all other population subgroups with whose values they may be incompatible.

The question of choice is central to the ethical evaluation of public health programmes. Is the choice informed by full disclosure of its advantages and disadvantages? Is the population of subjects free to refuse to participate? Do all have equal access to the means for making a choice of recommended patterns of diet, exercise, stress avoidance, and the like?

Methods of behaviour control, as exemplified by child rearing practices, are ubiquitous in every society. However, behaviour control in the modern sense refers to programmes designed on the basis of operant conditioning theory – that is, the manipulation of behaviour by controlling the contingencies of reinforcement. When a troubled patient seeks behaviour therapy to rid himself of unwanted symptoms, then he is a voluntary participant in an activity chosen in search of relief. This must be contrasted with attempts to modify the behaviour of populations who may not be seeking help and who have in any event not given informed consent. Particular problems arise in the case of 'captive' populations, such as prisoners, the institutionalised mentally ill, the incompetent elderly, the mentally retarded.

There are those who advocate changing behaviour by aversion methods – for example, making smokers or drinkers individually responsible for the health consequences of their behaviour by means of higher premiums on insurance policies or by refusal of coverage. How far can such proposals be considered ethical if medical knowledge suggests that these health damaging behaviours represent addictions rather than the personal failure to make a proper moral choice?

When parents fail to provide adequate nurture for their children, how far is the state warranted in intervening in order to promote the health of the child? Most societies accept that principle in the instance of physical abuse. Does it apply to emotional and cognitive abuse? What are the consequences for the integrity of the family if society intervenes too readily, however laudable its goals?

Finally, are there times of crisis in society which warrant the overriding of freedom of choice in the name of common survival? This issue can be illustrated in terms of the population crises which faces the People's Republic of China. Is a 'one-child family' policy enforced through social sanctions and even compulsory abortion a legitimate response to the threat of an ecological disaster if the present birth rate continues?

DR DOXIADIS

Regarding randomised controlled trials, it is, I think, important to remember that health raises many ethical questions. We cannot simply say that every health programme or policy decision must be the subject of a randomised controlled trial before it can be put into operation. Other ethical dilemmas may intrude and each case is likely to be different.

Dr Eisenberg makes the point that there is a contrast between the request by an individual for help in changing his behaviour in order to relieve his symptoms and health modification programmes addressed to population groups. Population groups are in fact already in many instances subjected to behaviour modification through the medium of commercial advertising. So it is not only the state or a health agency which tries to change behaviour.

The same argument can be applied to the point about aversion methods. Doctors in the normal one-to-one relationship with their patients use aversion methods, whether they realise it or not. When, for instance, a mother brings a very obese child to me, I try to explain why she should help the child to lose weight. I have to justify my advice by explaining the potential long-term risks of obesity. I have to stress the risks to the child's health, I have to make her afraid of something. This is a use of aversion methods. Again if a heavy smoker with the beginnings of emphysema goes to his family doctor, he will be advised to stop smoking because to continue will threaten his life. This too is a type of aversion therapy.

There is also a personal example of the use of aversion methods in health education which I would like to mention. Until 1980, Greece had an annual increase of six per cent in tobacco consumption. We then started a very intensive anti-smoking campaign and for almost three years, the annual rise fell to zero, a very important and rapid result. In order to achieve this, we used television advertisements which could be considered as aversive. A couple, for example, would be seen going to a cafeteria for a cup of coffee. As they sat down, one said to the other 'it is time for a cigarette' and a background voice said 'it is time for cancer'. This was considered very frightening, but we achieved a very important result. Unfortunately, with a change of government, the anti-smoking campaign stopped and the annual increase jumped to 10 per cent. Thus, I think it is legitimate, especially for those in clinical practice, to suggest the need for some use of aversion in trying to influence people's behaviour in relation to habits which damage their health.

Dr Eisenberg also raised the very important point of state intervention in the case of child abuse. It is perhaps obvious that the state should intervene in cases of physical abuse, and even in cases of emotional abuse, although this becomes more complex to judge. The issue of cognitive abuse, however, leads to very slippery ground and eventually to totalitarianism – what do we mean by cognitive abuse? In extreme cases of gross sensory deprivation, for example, intervention would certainly be required. But does the state have the right to intervene in cases where there is a cognitive abuse in the sense that the parents want to try and teach their child a certain set of values.

PROFESSOR GOROVITZ

Dr Eisenberg's mode of presentation is by raising questions rather than suggesting his views of what the answers should be. In discussing the question of choice, for example, he asks is the population of subjects free to refuse? In so far as this is a rhetorical question with an implied value that the answer should be 'yes' before an intervention can be justified, there are some difficulties. One of our central concerns is surely to determine the limits of justification for imposing measures where the subjects are not free to refuse. An example of this is in fluoridation of the water supply. In this case, the population is clearly not free to refuse, except in theory by the elaborate and costly method of developing an independent water supply. In general, I do not think we can accept the view that in every case, the population must be free to refuse. Where possible, I would prefer to see the question asked a little differently – do the merits of the case justify overriding the population's freedom to refuse?

Dr Eisenberg also asks whether all subjects have equal access to the means for making a choice, for example, on diet or exercise. Again that is an extremely stringent standard of justification. If we recommend certain diets, some people will be excluded from participating because of allergies or digestive problems. And it may be that some people cannot exercise because of cardiac conditions. If we impose a requirement of equal access absolutely strictly – that is, everyone in the population must have fully equal access to the recommended pattern of behaviour – we make impossible certain modes of intervention that would be beneficial to large portions of the population simply because we cannot extend them to the whole population.

Again, on the question of behaviour modification with respect to excessive use of alcohol or tobacco, we are offered the stark contrast between viewing these habits as addiction on the one hand or as a morally culpable free choice on the other. The distinction is not as clear as that and it is surely possible to view addictive behaviour as partly culpable. People can, for example, be encouraged with some success to try to develop a perspective on their own addictive behaviour and to cooperate in measures to free them from that addiction. Simply to say 'I am an addict' is an insufficient way of responding to criticism of a particular kind of self-damaging behaviour. The implicit suggestion here is that, if there is medical evidence that smoking in a particular individual is an addiction, it becomes entirely inappropriate to hold him responsible for his behaviour. This is surely an oversimplification.

Finally, I would like to say a word on cognitive abuse. The state does require that children be educated in accordance with standards determined not by the family but by some external constituencies. We have occasionally in the United States the situation in which a family decides that it wishes to educate its children independently, in ways that do not satisfy the state's requirements. The state can then intervene, viewing the family's behaviour as a kind of cognitive abuse. This is, I agree, a very dangerous and delicate issue but there is precedent for what the justifiable limits of such an intervention should be.

DISCUSSION

Discussants: Roy (Chairman), Beauchamp, Blaney, Campbell, Doxiadis, Gorovitz, Martin, Pinet, Sand, Strasser, Tatsis, Veatch, Zakopoulos

Discussion on Dr Eisenberg's presentation centred on the use of aversion methods and on the role of different mechanisms of society, such as education and government, in health.

In the opening comment on this section of the session it was suggested that aversion methods of changing behaviour are appropriate in those cases where the patient or subject requests the intervention. Dr Eisenberg seemed to be commenting on the use of aversion methods to change behaviour in cases where the subject's benefit is all that is at stake and the subject is not initiating a request for those changes. There are serious moral problems raised by that strategy, and it may be that Dr Eisenberg misunderstands the motivation behind those who have been proposing some of the things he suggests, such as different insurance premiums for smokers, drinkers, and the like. It is radically different to advocate intervention to change a person's behaviour for his own benefit on the one hand and on the other, to advocate intervention not to change behaviour, but simply to produce a fair accounting for the costs that are involved. The former is a form of paternalism, the latter is a form of promoting just distribution of cost.

If society undertakes aversion methods, for the purpose of benefiting individuals who are not requesting such changes, society becomes an advocate of a particular set of value trade-offs for individuals. It can be argued that that is not the business of society. This argument leads directly to the credo mentioned in Dr Strasser's presentation which implies that health professionals should become involved in a very strange debate in which health values are traded off against other values in society. The health professional then becomes an evangelist for a particular set of values. The extension of this is that advocates of low fat foods or of recreational lifestyles or indeed each set of professionals would advocate the advantages of their own particular value pattern. This puts the health professional into an evangelistic role quite different from his traditional activities, and has considerable implications.

This view was strongly countered as implying that the state possesses no purpose, no sense of a common or shared life. In liberal societies particularly, the notion of a community or shared sense of values of a common life is a difficult one because of the emphasis placed on individual freedom of choice. However, even in the most intensely liberal societies, such as the United States, there is still some sense of the Aristotelian notion of the community being formed for the common good. The community exists in part for the sake of providing for one another, for recognising each other as fellow members of a particular society, and for expressing some shared sense of values, among which in almost every democratic country, health is preeminent. Most liberal philosophers believe that by promoting the value of health, we create the ground for people to live out their own plan of life, to choose their own destiny.

There can be nothing wrong in health professionals advocating a healthy life for the population, unless we can object to people advocating the values that they believe in and identify with. It becomes more difficult when people are forced to choose a particular lifestyle, especially when this choice is made on a one-to-one basis. There is less difficulty with the use of coercion in society as a whole and we should not avoid the word. In a political community, coercion is a widely used, often abused, but legitimate way of expressing the common good.

The aversion method of dealing with health problems is based on a model of causation which attributes all of the causes of a particular illness or difficulty to the individual and his unhealthy lifestyle. This model may in fact be inappropriate to many of the matters under discussion. If we take the problem of alcohol dependency syndrome, for example, current epidemiological evidence suggests that the overall consumption and use of alcohol in society is one of the major aetiological factors in the development of alcoholism. We should at least examine this alternative model because its implications are entirely different. The fields for action are not against the individual in changing his behaviour, and imposing financial and other penalties for injuries incurred through his alcoholic behaviour. The action in this context is to be taken by the producers of alcohol and those who can devise methods for reducing or altering the patterns of distribution or consumption within society. These measures swing the responsibility away from the individual and on to government, public health authorities, and commercial interests, and a great deal of available epidemiological evidence supports that kind of approach.

As a reaction to aversion methods, it was also suggested that there might be some new orientation of health education towards more information and less education. But behaviour does not usually change simply through cold information and here positive conditioning may be more effective than aversive conditioning. General practitioners can play an important role in this context by entering real, honest dialogue with patients and families, listening and exchanging views, and providing advice based on accurate health facts.

Reference was made to a balanced and clear treatment of the role of doctors and other health professionals as health advocates in a recent book by Professor Nigel Stott, entitled Primary Health Care: Bridging the Gap between Theory and Practice.

We must beware also of a confusion between the term society and the term state. In many places around the world, the term society is used as an ideological cover-up for the state. Their purposes are frequently very different because the state is run by certain groups of people who change from time to time through elections or coups whereas society remains more constant. The state is often also assumed to be a rational organisation for the pursuit of specific goals and this is not the case in most states around the world. In certain so-called traditional societies, families can also pose the main obstacle to implementing social policy because they tend to pass on certain prejudices or superstitions which may hinder development in health policies.

The whole nature of health education must be much more fully explored. To speak of health education, for example, without discussing what education is, is not adequate. Education is not indoctrination and it is perfectly appropriate for the state to be concerned with health education, just as it is concerned with education as a whole. This is not an infringement of individual liberty.

The role of government must also be more fully examined in terms of its control of health destructive factors. Government has surely a clear task of control and coercion in regulating those adverse factors in advertising and in other aspects of our society which can be shown to be health destructive. This task is directly relevant to health education and is a very strong political responsibility that should be undertaken.

The health professions have a central role in the advocacy of health. The main theme of the World Health Organisation goal of health for all is intended to stress the importance of health as part of an overall strategy for society rather than as a marketable commodity.

CONCLUDING REMARKS

DR DOXIADIS

We have heard two main points of view on the reasons implicit in intervention on health or attempts at positive health education. One is that the government or health authority intervenes to influence and try to protect the individual who, by a particular habit or lifestyle, is damaging his health. The second is that such intervention is made not to protect the individual from the consequences of his behaviour but to make him accountable to society for the cost of that behaviour.

There is, however, a third factor which is extremely important and which has not been mentioned and that is the damage caused by a particular lifestyle to a third party. The children of smoking parents, for example, have double the incidence of respiratory infections than those whose parents do not smoke. At the age of 11 years these children are also six to seven months behind in tests of reading ability and arithmetic. Thus there are even more important long-term effects. Furthermore, non-smoking wives of smoking husbands have a higher incidence of lung cancer.

This changes the picture a little when we consider the rationale behind efforts to influence the habits of the smoking father. We now have another motivation to try and encourage him to stop smoking – not for the sake of his own health, not to make him realise the true cost to society of the consequent illnesses he will suffer, but because his lifestyle is damaging his immediate environment and the health of those close to him. Finally, a court in Sweden has recently ruled that passive smoking and its negative effects can be classified as an occupational injury. The relatives of a woman who had never smoked but who died of lung cancer because she had worked in close contact with six chain smoking colleagues for 18 years, obtained the above ruling. This is, therefore, another important factor to be considered.

ETHICAL ISSUES IN THE ACTIVITIES OF MASS MEDIA COMMUNICATION IN HEALTH EDUCATION

CLAIRE RAYNER

HOLLY WOOD HOUSE, HARROW-ON-THE-HILL

PROFESSOR GOROVITZ (CHAIRMAN)

The first paper of Session VI is by another speaker in absentia, Claire Rayner, an experienced freelance journalist and broadcaster. Dr Richard Nicholson will present the paper on her behalf and will include some comments and examples of his own. We are delighted also to have with us for this session a representative of the mass communication media in Greece and well-known author, Mr Nicos Dimou.

DR NICHOLSON FOR CLAIRE RAYNER

I was a little sad at one point to realise that thus far we have had really very little discussion related to our host nation, Greece. So I thought I would open by reading some comments on health preservation as applied to Greece from an example of the mass media.

'The general rules of health to be observed in Greece are similar to those required in south Italy and other southern lands. The visitor should invariably be somewhat more warmly clad than in a similar temperature at home and he should never leave the house without an overcoat to be donned on passing from sunshine to shade, when sitting in a boat or carriage, and in the evening. The sun is so strong even in winter that the difference of temperature in the shade is very marked. In cooler seasons the traveller should avoid sitting in the shade, especially on the cold stones of ruined buildings. It is also necessary to be warmly covered during sleep, the supply of bedclothes of the hotels and lodging houses is apt to be scanty. Catching cold is often a much more serious affair than in cooler climates and the first symptoms should be carefully attended to. Malarial fever is endemic only in a few of the low lying plains, such as those of Boatia, Argos, Laconia, and Delos, and generally manifests itself in the form of ague. Travellers who take sufficient nourishment and observe the most ordinary precautions are much less likely to suffer from it than the poorly fed, badly housed natives. They should be on their guard against the vapours rising from the ground after heavy rain and should avoid the evening, night, and early morning air as much as possible, especially when fasting. A moderate of spirits is said to be prophylactic against fever and quinine and change of air are the best cures.'

There are some further derogatory comments about the local inns. 'The traveller must bring his own coverings with him as the rugs presented him for bed clothes are almost always full of vermin. The pests which render night hideous include not only the flea, with which a traveller in Italy has probably become more or less familiar, but also bed bugs, lice and other disgusting insects, winged and wingless. The best remedies against the attacks of these enemies of repose is good insect powder, Persian or Keating, which should be plentifully sprinkled on the traveller's clothes and bedding.'

It is perhaps slightly unfair to read out of the 1894 edition of Baedeker's Advice to Travellers, particularly in view of the outstanding hospitality we are enjoying here in 1985. But in 1894 the written word was the only form of mass communication. Since then we have increased substantially the number of ways in which we can disseminate information and Claire Rayner, in her paper, has listed the various different possibilities.

It is very important that we consider the place of the mass media in preventive medicine. In much of our discussion so far, the assumption has been that the doctors or health professionals are going to do most of the work in health promotion and education. This is not in fact the case. A survey undertaken in Paris in the late 1970s, for example, showed that 47 per cent of Parisians regarded the mass media as their main source of health information with only 31 per cent seeking such information from health professionals.

Claire Rayner defines mass communication media as covering newspapers, magazines, television, radio, cinema, and video. She mentions also the role of live theatre which, although it has a smaller audience range, is attended by people who could be called opinion formers and also frequently feeds the wider media. There have been a number of interesting plays in Britain in recent years which fall into this category. 'Whose Life Is It Anyway' considered the question of whether an individual who is paralysed from the neck downwards has the right to demand to be allowed to die. 'Children of a Lesser God' provided a vivid insight into what life is really like for a deaf person.

The example of live radio phone-in programmes as a source of information will be questioned by some who might contend that they are more often a source of misinformation. But there are certainly radio programmes which provide a great deal of very useful information. One good example from the United Kingdom is a programme called 'The Archers' which has been broadcast daily for 30 or 40 years and has a large number of faithful listeners. Initially, soon after the Second World War, it disseminated information about developing agricultural methods and improving nutrition. More recently, it has been helpful in health education matters – on one occasion, various members of the cast were going to donate blood and there was subsequently a phenomenal increase in the number of blood donors nationwide. So radio can have quite an impact. Television can have an even greater impact. Claire Rayner uses the example of just how much damage is done when a popular comedian lights up a cigarette on a programme.

Through virtually all the activities of these different segments of the media – feature material, news, advertising, opinion or advice columns – information about health can be communicated.

Claire Rayner also describes how she believes the public sees public health as having two main components. First, there is what 'they' – that is, the health professionals – can do for you, in the way of immunisation, or running infant welfare clinics or screening services. And secondly, there is what you can do for yourself, by controlling the use of tobacco, alcohol or other drugs, by taking exercise, or by using natural herbal remedies. It is worth looking at some of the problems that do arise, particularly between health professionals and representatives of the media. One example of the conflict that can exist is the campaign against whooping cough immunisation in Great Britain. This was conducted initially by one newspaper with considerable support from one particular professor of community medicine, and it had a most dramatic effect. The uptake of whooping cough immunisation dropped in one year from 80 per cent to 30 per cent, and in 10 years since then it has only slowly crept up to somewhere between 48 and 50 per cent. So this one campaign, based on information from one doctor, which he sincerely believes but which no one else agrees with, has had this dramatic and damaging effect and probably resulted in at least 30 or 40 excess deaths of infants from whooping cough in the last decade in the United Kingdom.

A parallel problem arose in the United States in 1976 when the swine flu affair developed. In that case, it was found that when a mass immunisation programme against swine influenza was started, one in 100 000 people receiving the immunisation developed *Guillain-Barré* syndrome, polyneuropathy. That was perhaps considerably less important than the possible side-effects of whooping cough but there was a similar risk, in terms of probability. And the existence of that one in 100 000 risk of *Guillain-Barré* syndrome was enough to start a media campaign which led to a rapid presidential decision to cut off the whole of the immunisation programme when it was only about half completed.

Claire Rayner in her paper asks whether the status quo between health professionals and members of the media is satisfactory or whether there is need for some tightening of controls, some form of censorship. On the whole I think most people would agree that there is no place for censorship whatsoever, but that there is need of an improvement in communication. This can be amplified by another example from the United Kingdom. A few years ago a television programme was shown which examined the criteria for brain death. This left a very strong impression that transplant surgeons, in their anxiety for material, were removing kidneys from people before they were truly dead. At that time many doctors in the United Kingdom were so completely disgusted with that programme that they vowed never to speak to representatives of the media again. It seems to me that this is totally the wrong approach. If something goes wrong on a programme, if misinformation is transmitted in this way, there must obviously be some system of ensuring that the correct information can later be presented. The sort of debate and publicity that will ensue is probably ultimately of more value in health education than a simple published correction which cannot be seen as a media event. A properly conducted debate can be of great value. And, while it may be unrealistic to press for an automatic right of reply in the media when incorrect information is presented, there does need to be a greater willingness on the part of journalists and editors to give space or time for correction and for debate.

There is an interesting and worthwhile suggestion that it might be possible to set up a bureau of health professionals and experts to whom journalists could apply to obtain correct information on a particular subject, and this should perhaps be explored. In the United States, the Hastings Centre has reported recently that it had helped the local school of journalism in running courses to educate journalists about basic medical and medical ethical information. This is surely an area in which there is the possibility of doing far more.

The need for a code of ethics for journalists is also raised and it may be that overall there is a place for such a code. I do not think, however, that this should be related specifically to medical ethics. It should be part of a general code that applies to all media work with the central ethical problem to what extent are they representing the truth and to what extent are they attempting to represent the truth? There should undoubtedly be far greater and better collaboration between health professionals and members of the media to try to ensure the presentation of correct information and also to suggest sources of alternative information from those in the profession who may hold a different point of view.

I would like to add one point, not something I have discussed with Claire Rayner, but which relates to another educative effect of the mass media and which concerns us all. In the last few months in the United Kingdom, we have been exposed on television and in the newspapers to detailed coverage of the horrific effects of famine in Ethiopia. In previous times this sort of immediate information was not available and people were not aware of such difficulties. There is the case of the Irish potato famine in 1846 when, because the British people were not informed about the situation, the Government was able to ignore the problem and provide very little help for at least a year. It is something for which the British Government has been castigated ever since. We are now in a position to know what is happening in the developing world. We know that somewhere between three and five million children annually die of measles which could be prevented by a single injection. In the United Kingdom we would have to go back about 50 years to find a cumulative total of 1000 deaths from measles and subacute sclerosing panencephalitis. But, although we have information about a really severe current health problem, we seem to be content both in this meeting and in general in our medical communities in the western world to do very little about it.

We have seen in the last few months the effect of mass media coverage of famine in Ethiopia and other parts of Africa. The response from the general public has been a great deal swifter and more substantial than the response from governments. There is a feeling among the general public, which may not be shared by the medical profession, that we have a duty to do far more in the way of preventive medicine in developing countries than we are trying to do at the moment. This is, in my view, the most important problem in preventive health in the world today. How do we get the simple means of prevention, which we have known about and applied for years, to the places where they are needed? We in the western world have the resources, the money, and the technology. Yet somehow we seem to believe that our duties to other human beings extend only as far as our national borders. In a group like this, I suggest that we have a duty to examine this problem and be in a position to advise the EEC and NATO on how we can start trying to tackle it.

DISCUSSION

Discussants: Gorovitz (Chairman), Campbell, Canosa, Crawshaw, Dimou, Doxiadis, Dunstan, Karhausen, Riis, Roy, Tatsis, Tognoni, Violaki, Zander

The question of censorship was raised and it was suggested that this is a rather emotive term which implies something that most people would automatically mistrust and fear. Control may be a more appropriate word in this context and the control of the health detrimental and the health enhancing effects of the media is something that could be profitably examined.

In countries where medicine is not yet very much a matter of state authority, there is also a commercial point that is very relevant to ethics. In Greece, for example, it is not uncommon for doctors to give a press conference on specific issues with the sole aim of promoting their own name and have succeeded in this way in building up a lucrative private practice. The same method is adopted by medical companies to promote different drugs. A good relationship with a journalist, for example, can result in a five-column article on the wonder drug X which cures cancer, the worst kind of health information possible. This is an important ethical issue and an area where the medical profession should be very strict.

Health professionals, and perhaps particularly doctors, should also be much more courageous, frank, and informative in dealing with the media. The better we communicate, the smaller the risk of being misinterpreted. There is an important distinction between informing and elaborating information. It is the job of the media to inform but there is a danger in elaborating on specialised information without a detailed training and knowledge of the subject. Anyone can inform, for example, about the famine in Africa but elaboration of the health or nutritional aspects of the problem should be confined to a health professional. In Spain, for example, one of the most popular current television programmes, called 'Better to Prevent' is presented by a lawyer although it deals with matters such as breastfeeding, vitamins, and family planning. It may be more satisfactory if professional people stick to their own particular professional business.

As far as a code of ethics is concerned, journalism, in common with every profession, does have such a code. The problem with codes of ethics is that they are usually wishful thinking and serve mainly to project an optimal image of the profession. Ethics requires practical, day-to-day collaboration between the media and the medical profession so that misinterpretation and misinformation can be avoided or at least minimised. About 80 per cent of media errors or misinformation are not deliberate but stem from a lack of knowledge and understanding of medical matters on the part of journalists. They may receive a good, clear statement from a doctor or from a health authority. They then translate this in their own terms and errors of fact or emphasis occur.

The mass communication media has of course responsibility for negative or positive coverage of health matters. But even here there are conflicts. How do we equate, for example, an excellent programme on nutrition for schools with the very persuasive advertising of so-called junk foods which children can hardly avoid seeing on television. There has to be reliable collaboration between responsible people from various professions in this as in any other field. As an example of irresponsibility, there was at one stage in Greece a news story about a new method of treating cancer with the water of Camaterosa, as it was called. And although it was discredited by the High Supreme Health Council, people continued to seek this kind of treatment with a sort of hysterical faith because of media coverage and advertisement.

One of the outcomes of the Oregon Health Decisions project was a very strong resolution that the media should have their own meeting in which they would examine their ethical stance. In the field of prevention it was discovered that in the current Oregon health delivery system, organ transplantation was not undertaken. There are, however, people who need livers and hearts. They turn to the press for publicity in order to alert the public to the fact that, for example, a child, whose life could be saved at a cost of $50 000, is going to die of biliary atresia. This kind of mass hysteria has occurred repeatedly, despite the fact that the reporters were given very adequate information about the trade-offs and about why it was not felt that the state should be paying for highly technical manouevres when so much preventive health work remained to be done. And the reporters again and again had difficulty with their editors. The editors would take the story, look at what would sell the paper, and remove all the information that gave the real sense of choice that the community had to face.

So we must provide journalists with sufficient backing from the medical profession to stand up responsibly to their editors – to say, for example, if you are going to run this story, you must include not only the details of the personal death or loss that is going to occur but also the information that goes with it relative to the whole community. If misinformation is presented there is also the possibility of replying by a different route – for example, by using the medical journals to publish a responsible correction.

Claire Rayner's paper rather assumes a fairly stable social situation without rapid technological advance and implies that the mechanisms that have worked, perhaps particularly in Britain, so far, to encourage reasonable presentation and balanced argument, will somehow continue to do so. We must look more carefully at the revolution in communication technology – developments in areas such as cable television and microcomputers – and the implications of this for the relationship between the media and health professionals and for the whole idea of control. The power of television was emphasised and attention drawn to the importance of using this particular medium in countries where other forms of mass communication, such as newspapers, are distributed or used as sources of information by a very small proportion of the population. In a poll of people in Greece exposed to an active television campaign on various aspects of health education, it was found that over 90 per cent of those interviewed had absorbed some information on matters such as dental health, obesity, childhood accidents, and so on.

The paper also addresses only one aspect of the subject – the information-carrying responsibility of the public media. There is another important aspect which is much more difficult to analyse and that is expressive power. This is not a purely rhetorical statement because this question has been causing a great deal of anxiety, particularly in the United States, to child psychiatrists, sociologists, and paediatricians. There is some strong evidence that part of the new juvenile criminality might be attributable to the internalisation of the violence shown in the cinema or on television at peak viewing hours. This is in contrast to the previous tradition of literature, of theatre, of cinema which showed criminality as something out there, not something inside our daily lives. There is a danger that children internalise violence as an accepted form of behaviour and it becomes a pattern of living. Some attention should, therefore, be paid to the impact of the expressive aspect of the public media in contrast to its information-carrying role and the ethical questions this raises.

Another aspect of concern for which the media is largely responsible is the exporting of certain prototypes of behaviour from one context to another where they may not be appropriate. An example of this is in the aerobic exercise programme of Jane Fonda which has achieved massive coverage and popularity in many countries. The programme, however, can lead to unrealistic expectations and psychological strains in those who are unable to achieve an image perceived as desirable. It can also of course result in considerable physical damage.

A cautious approach was recommended to the suggestion of establishing an advice or information bureau, at least so far as smaller countries are concerned. There is a more flexible and cheaper model, which already operates in Denmark, for example, in which a number of influential and respected doctors or specialists act as mediators and advisers to the media. They do not give answers to specific questions but can provide the names of specialists on the subject in question. In the United States there is an organisation which exists strictly for making referrals of this sort. The Bureau on Science and the Media has a register of some thousands of scientists specialising in a full range of subjects and serves as a referral source for the responsible media.

An advisory board could also be a regulatory body, consisting of members of the press and doctors, which would have power to regulate all matters pertaining to health information. This formula has been tried in fields other than medicine and it has worked. In Britain, for example, there is the Advertising Council where members of the press, the media, and advertising agencies have a regulatory function. Such a bureau should under no circumstances belong to the medical profession. To leave control in the hands of a few established representatives of the profession would run the risk of inhibiting rather than expediting the development of a better relationship with the media. It must belong to those who want to use it and its usage and efficacy will depend on the contribution we are prepared to make.

The media is of course a well-established profession and all our words of control and advice are perhaps somewhat unrealistic. The health professions cannot actually control the media nor is there any reason why they should. To expect journalists to adhere to certain codes of practice appropriate in the medical context is neither possible nor necessarily desirable. We need to examine much more critically our own responsibility towards ensuring either that appropriate health information is carried in the media, and to what extent we can cooperate to ensure that television programmes, for example, present medical topics accurately and responsibly. There are instances where this has happened in Britain. The College of General Practitioners undertook a series of 14 television programmes on preventive care where there was a partnership between the profession and the people producing the programme. And before preaching to the media about a possible code of ethics, the medical profession must surely try to clarify its own slightly confused ethical code and ambivalent attitude to the media. There is a very definite ethical part of our code in the United Kingdom concerning advertising. Many doctors are still reluctant to appear on television in case it can be in some way construed as a form of advertising. There is a great deal of confusion about this and we do need to clarify the ethics involved. We need to think very creatively not only about the contribution the media can make to improving information on health but also how we can constructively contribute to the media.

Finally, Dr Nicholson was congratulated for drawing attention to the appalling health and hunger problems of the developing world. We must try to move into a global framework for preventive medicine and it may be appropriate to devote some space in the publications that will result from our current work to this question. The terms of reference of medical ethics are constantly changing and the medical profession cannot afford simply to observe. Whether we like it or not, in the modern world, the medical profession has got to acknowledge its collective responsibility for factors such as preventable disease or hunger in the developing world. If we do not face up to these issues, which lie partly in the field of international politics, and the profession itself is split about this kind of commitment, we risk losing our credibility and the confidence of the public.

CONCLUDING REMARKS

DR NICHOLSON

I would like to say briefly that I was grateful for the points made on the extension of our concern to the developing countries. The provision of preventive health techniques to these countries, where 70 per cent of the population has no access to even routine immunisation, is a major ethical problem and a matter of the highest priority.

ETHICAL ISSUES IN OCCUPATIONAL HEALTH

EDWARD POCHIN

NATIONAL RADIOLOGICAL PROTECTION BOARD, CHILTON, DIDCOT, OXFORDSHIRE

PROFESSOR GOROVITZ (CHAIRMAN)

It is a great pleasure to introduce the next speaker, Sir Edward Pochin. Sir Edward is Consultant to the Director of the National Radiological Protection Board and has over 30 years of involvement in radiation protection and concern with radiation risks. After his paper there will be a short presentation by Professor Rainer Muller of the University of Bremen.

SIR EDWARD POCHIN

It is, I believe, quite essential in any review of occupational risk, to try to be quantitative about the size of the risk involved as well as being descriptive about its nature. Any examination of the safety or risk of different occupations makes it immediately clear that it is not the case that there are some safe occupations and other hazardous occupations. All occupations involve some risk. There is a continuous spectrum through existing occupations. They all involve some risks, even of fatal occupational accidents, risks imposed by the nature of the work, the working conditions, staffing, management, equipment, and so on. This opens up a whole new territory of ethical problems which we have not had the opportunity to touch on so far.

There is a tendency to think in rather black and white terms about ethical obligations. It is perceived as ethically wrong to condone or imply or allow an imposed risk, any risk, certainly any substantial risk. Yet in fact, the risks at work, even quite simply of accidental death from injury, from working causes, range in the United Kingdom from three deaths per million at risk per year to 3000 deaths per million at risk per year in conventional everyday industries: boots and shoes and making of clothing, three deaths per million per year (estimated quite accurately wth a standard error of about one, on 22 years averaged experience in a working population of about half a million), up to something like 3000 per million at risk – a thousand times as many – in fishing at sea, trawling and accidental death there. So far this is straightforward. We try to lower these accident risks as effectively as possible. There are figures available on the percentage reduction of such risks per year, generally falling two, three, four, five per cent, occasionally up to 10 per cent of their value per year over time.

But the position becomes much more difficult where we are not just deciding the risks that are acceptable in conventional industries where no risk is acceptable if it can be lowered. It is even more difficult to decide the risks of chemical or physical agents, like radiation, in the working environment; and specially difficult, if there is no threshold level of exposure to those chemicals or radiation below which the exposure is completely safe. If we have to assume that the risk may extend right down to zero, then we have a real problem. How low must the risk be to be recommended as acceptable, if some risk must be accepted? I take radiation as an example because of the mass of reliable human epidemiological data of the risks from given doses of radiation and the very extensive radiobiological work ranging over a period of 50 years on the effects of ionising radiation.

This illustrates a whole host of ethical questions. First of all, how do we compare different kinds of risk – the risks of accidental death, accidental injuries, radiation-caused cancers, radiation-induced genetic effects? How can risks be aggregated to permit comparison of an occupation with risks from chemicals or radiation and from injuries, with an occupation where the injuries predominate? Clearly this involves two steps. First, the clinical or scientific step of making the best possible assessment of the risk of death, or of death and injury if they can be aggregated. This is the technical assessment of the amount or size of the risk.

The second step is to obtain a population assessment of the amount of weight attached by the community to different kinds of injury or damage. In terms of death, for example, there will be a difference in the weight attached to an accidental and immediate death from falling off a ladder, and a radiation exposure which may induce a cancer which will only appear in 25 to 30 years time. How can we compare the balance between the immediate and 'clean' type of accidental death and the more ugly and insidious form of death from a disease which develops over time? This requires an opinion from an informed population, an informed community – and by that I mean a technically informed community, and not, with respect, a television informed community – on the size of the risks. I think this is dangerous because I am coming near to asking for a sort of technical dictatorship which must be categorical about the size of the risk; but this population should also be informed sufficiently to say how it views different types of risk. Essentially this has to be a probability evaluation as to the importance of different risks. This raises a very interesting general point for discussion because, for example, the cancers and genetic effects induced by radiation are indistinguishable, microscopically or in their nature and clinical behaviour, from cancers or genetic effects that occur naturally. So the distinction is not with the microscope, it is with statistics.

In terms of compensation in the event of a development of a cancer, we have to consider numerically the probability that the cancer may have been caused by chemicals or radiation, compared with the probability that it arose from natural causes. Certainly the legal profession in Britain is not very much at home with numerical differences in the weight to be attached to the occupational risk and the natural risk, and such an evaluation does cause problems.

If we allow ourselves to be guided by popular information without the technical knowledge of an informed community, we will tend to treat anxieties rather than deaths. We will take steps to reduce popular anxiety – and anxiety is just as anxious if it is misinformed. Some anxieties can be worse than death, as the fact that people commit suicide because of oppressive anxieties shows. In general, an informed public should be able to attach weights to the different types of risk which are evaluated technically. And here the quantification of risk and the balance between quantifiable risk and quantifiable benefit quite clearly spill over into medicine. The archaic medical principle, *primum non nocere*, dates from the time when most medical remedies conferred very little benefit on their recipients and so it was important to ensure that at least they did no harm. In the modern context, that is a rather timid medical attitude. To achieve the probability of curing certain severe diseases it is nowadays sometimes necessary to advocate remedies which themselves carry some risk. And we have to be certain that the risk they carry is less, and considerably less, than the benefits that they confer.

These are the points that I would like to stress. The medical situation is a very uncomfortable one when we are asked as clinicians to propose a course of treatment which involves some hazard in the pursuit of a greater good. It becomes even more uncomfortable when we attempt to give informed guidance to the patient or to his family as to the risks and obtain informed consent to a procedure or operation. If the procedure or operation in question is one that carries a one per cent risk of death at the time of the operation, what do we say? We can say that the risk is small; but if we say honestly and factually that it is one per cent, then that particular patient will be that one per cent during the next five sleepless nights.

There is thus a whole set of serious and difficult ethical questions which arise in the occupational context and which spill over in their relationship to clinical medicine.

SUBSIDIARY PRESENTATION

ROLE OF THE COMPANY PHYSICIAN

RAINER MÜLLER

UNIVERSITY OF BREMEN, BREMEN

I would like to express a few thoughts about the ethical questions which, in my own experience, arise in occupational medicine, and relate this particularly to the role of the company physician.

The company physician works in a situation with a high level of social conflict. The health interests of the employee are not identical with the productivity interests of the employer. The duty of the company physician is merely to advise management in legal terms, his function is to reduce the liability of the employer for accidents and for occupational diseases. He is not a member of a governmental health and safety administration, and he has no legal right to intervene for safer workplace conditions. The role of the company doctor and his relationship to the employee, therefore, cannot be compared with a typical doctor-patient relationship in primary health care. Job seekers or employees do not usually go to him of their own free will. We cannot speak of a confidential relationship. In formal terms, the company doctor is responsible primarily to the employer, and only indirectly to the interests of the employee by preventing or reducing health risks. But, as a result of his diagnosis, he may cause social damage to his patient, the employee, in terms of unemployment, loss of income, or loss of a familiar workplace. The company doctor frequently has little or no control over the social consequences of his diagnostic decision.

With regard to his activities, there is no unity of diagnosis, therapy, or primary prevention in respect to the problem of exposure to risk. The centre of his activities is not to uncover pathogenic working conditions but rather to examine job seekers or employees. The opinion of a company doctor on the health of an individual is used by non-medical people outside the medical system, to make employment and personnel decisions. The confidentiality of personal data about a patient cannot be guaranteed.

Physicians, as well as doctors working in occupational medicine, are trained in a patient-centred and disease-centred tradition. The inclusion of environmental aspects in the medical training is grossly underdeveloped and many doctors have no knowledge in this field. Systematic recognition of workplace hazards is also neglected in regard to the classical chemical and physical agents, and where any notice of these problems is taken, it tends to be concentrated on a single factor. Scientific knowledge is curiously deficient concerning facts about combined hazards, particularly if they include psychological and social stress. Little knowledge exists about long-term effects.

State and accident insurance regulations stipulate more and more health criteria for employment in specific occupations. Analytical procedures of diagnosis, such as gene screening and biological monitoring, increasingly enable recognition of susceptibilities of particular employees at an early stage. With modern techniques of epidemiology, mass screening, and information technology, the profiles of workplace requirements can be compared with the performance, fitness, and qualifications of employees and job seekers. The company doctor supplies the necessary data and the management uses this information to select suitable personnel, as well as for the rationalisation and intensification of work.

Epidemiological research is also involved in turning the principle of public health on its head. In research carried out in my department, for example, we have analysed personal data from health insurances over a period of years. The results of these studies revealed the possibility of making a prognosis concerning the interrelationships of constellations of social variables with the probable development of chronic diseases. It is possible to use these epidemiological profiles with prognostic possibilities for personnel policies within companies. They can also be used in preventive medicine to determine or identify populations at risk.

There is, in West Germany and elsewhere, increasing use of microelectronic information systems and the storing of enormous amounts of personal data on social, economic, and medical factors in companies and social security offices. Physicians and doctors in occupational health provide data for this with wider implications for medicine in general and for occupational medicine specifically. It can lead, for example, to the separation of diagnosis from health care, the transformation of therapeutic activity to mere assessment, the subordination of medical experts to the interests of bureaucracy and business. These are some of the ethical issues in this field which deserve our attention.

DISCUSSION

Discussants: Gorovitz (Chairman), Blaney, Crawshaw, Jeanneret, Knox, Pinet, Riis, Roy, Strasser

This was felt to be another area in which an international view on prevention and the ethics of prevention is extremely important. Occupational hazards which are expensive to eliminate, for example, can result in a company moving its operations from a country with strict health and safety regulations to another where these issues are not regarded as important. The hazards remain but employees and the community are not protected. Equally, the damaging effects of the sulphur dioxide emitted in one country may be transported to another by prevailing winds. It is thus extremely important to have an international viewpoint.

The recurring ethical dilemma of the need for research and information and the protection of the individual's right to privacy and confidentiality does arise in a particular way in occupational health. It is certainly very much to the fore in the Federal Republic of Germany and there is a current clash on data collection on cancer which requires a multidisciplinary approach. The problem of confidentiality in the field of data storage by computer is particularly difficult because, whatever the safeguards, it is possible to break into most filing systems. The possible solution of keeping the individual identification data and the health data apart has its own inherent dangers. There have been cases where the state has threatened to close a data collection centre unless procedures were revised to comply with the basic requirements for data protection.

After these initial comments, discussion centred on the inevitability of risk-taking and the quantification of risks. As Sir Edward rightly stressed, we must accept that no work can be without risk and no treatment without risk. This is a sound basis on which to approach the subject because there is a common belief that there are risk-free treatments and working conditions.

So what kind of information are we going to give the individual? When we collect data on occupational groups it is possible to say that there is a one per cent risk per year in a particular job of having an accident at work. But what about the individual worker preparing to go through an operation? We cannot hide behind percentages in the clinical situation. We must try to translate that one per cent into a meaningful statement for the patient, weighing the risks and benefits in an understandable way and trying to place ourselves as clinicians in the patient's place.

If we extend the concept of risk-taking outside of the occupational sphere into general risk-taking for society as a whole, we can see that epidemiological studies have shown that risk may be quite low for some things and quite high for others. On the question of breast cancer, for example, it is known that having a baby late in life only increases the risk of the disease by two. Working in the deep sea fishing industry, on the other hand, involves a risk of death of 3000 per million exposed per year or even more. Cigarette smokers have a risk of illness or death about 20 or 30 times greater than non-smokers.

One of the issues we must examine is where does our ethical duty to intervene come along the risk spectrum? At what point do we have an ethical duty to intervene, at what size of risk is it ethical to intervene? This may be a question without an answer but we must try to decide. This whole question of quantification of risk is very important. In interpreting the results of intervention trials, for example, it is really essential to try to quantify the risks identified to provide a sound basis for implementation of the results. So what level of risk is it reasonable to ignore, what is a negligible risk? As soon as we realise that everything has some risk, this becomes a compulsory question. Different professions approach this question in different ways. Physicists, for example, go in for numerology. They produce figures based on integral numbers of standard errors, and on this basis provide the advice that you can double the risk or you can accept the risk that people in Aberdeen accept because they live in granite houses with radiation. But these definitions of negligible risk do not work in the real world.

Eventually we might have to conclude that a negligible risk is a risk which is neglected. It is a behavioural definition, not something that can be imposed externally. If we want to define a negligible risk, we have to observe people and see what risk they neglect or ignore. These people have to be informed about the risk and it has to be a risk to them and not to someone else. And, of course, the first thing we find in doing this is a high degree of inconsistency. There are some quite high risks which people do neglect and there are some very low risks which they do not. It is possible to produce an informed scale of description of behaviour. In an experiment on this, the smallest risk found which people did not neglect was phenylketonuria in the newborn, which has a risk of about 1 in 20 000 births and for which there is a routine screening test. This can then serve as a reference level of the lowest risk that people do not neglect. Thus, if we wish to define a negligible risk it can only usefully be done in behavioural terms and presented as a behavioural definition.

We must also try to decide whose duty it is to intervene. In clinical medicine, the answer is clear: it is the duty of the individual doctor to provide his patient with information about risks and to give advice. But in public health and preventive medicine, the situation is altogether more complex. Who is responsible, for example, for deaths from asbestosis? It is easy to single out the employer as culprit but does this exonerate the medical profession? Can we point the finger at television and say this television programme – such as the one referred to earlier which disrupted kidney transplant work to a regrettable extent – has caused this many deaths? The question of whose is the duty is very complex but its complexity does not exonerate us from responsibility. Should we in fact be trying to do more to identify those responsible for unacceptable risks in the occupational field and take appropriate measures against them?

CONCLUDING REMARKS

SIR EDWARD POCHIN

In response to Professor Muller's comment and in particular on his point about long-term effects, I would say this. One of the difficulties of chemical assessment is that there are so many chemicals emerging each year that there is very little chance of assessing their long-term effects individually. With radiation, on the other hand, the only important effects of low doses are long-term ones and that should be a warning.

Coming to the general discussion, the radiation field is perhaps fortunate in having an international forum of the sort suggested. There is an International Commission on Radiological Protection which commands a healthy balance of respect and disrespect. It is composed of 70 or 80 highly competent scientists from about 25 countries, meeting regularly and publishing reports.

On the point about conflict between data collection and privacy, a working group, a work force, will, I think, tend to be happier to agree to the study of causes of death in an attempt to establish the safety or hazards of their occupation than of the causes of current disease in individuals, which is obviously a more sensitive area.

On the question of assessment and quantification of risks, excellent points were made. On the risk from cigarette smoking, one can either say that three-quarters of one cigarette will give you a one in a million risk of dying from smoking or that each cigarette will cost you, proportionally, seven minutes of life expectancy. Finally, on negligible risk, I agree that it is not the job of physicists or of physicians to discuss what people regard as negligible. What we have to do is to go outside the committee room and see what people actually accept or neglect. What I would hope is that the group whose opinions are sought – and some funny groups have been analysed by people studying this question of perceived risk – will be making its decision not only on the kind of risk, but also on the size of risk involved.

ETHICS, PREVENTION, AND CHILD HEALTH

ALFRED SAND

DEPARTMENT OF PUBLIC HEALTH, FREE UNIVERSITY OF BRUSSELS, BRUSSELS

DR NICHOLSON (CHAIRMAN)

Our first speaker this session is Professor Alfred Sand from the School of Public Health at the Université Libre in Brussels. Professor Sand began his medical career as a general practitioner and then became a paediatrician and child psychiatrist. He is now involved in research on psychosocial health issues, particularly in the fields of child development, family health, and mental health.

PROFESSOR SAND

I propose to discuss ethics, prevention, and child health and add some remarks about mental health issues and prevention which are perhaps among the most difficult questions to tackle in the field of ethics. First some basic comments about paediatrics, prevention, and ethics. Many of the rules that apply to paediatrics are similar to those applied to clinical practice among adults. But there are exceptions to this statement of which the question of informed consent is a very relevant example, in view of its ethical implications. What should be the criteria of age, or IQ, or mental age which allow us to ask the child for his consent to some research or preventive procedure?

Another fundamental point is that research on adults, whether in prevention or not, cannot replace research on children in all cases. A good example here is immunisation, where effective research will require a child population. Thus, whether we like the idea of research involving children or not, it has to be done and done quite extensively for many health problems.

I would like to look now at a few specific preventive measures and the ethical problems which may arise from them. My co-author, Manciaux, and myself place great emphasis on the declaration on the rights of children, les Droits de l'Enfant. Principle 8 of this declaration contains the statement that 'the child should, in all circumstances, be among the first ones to receive protection and care'. We shall see that unfortunately this is not always the case.

The obvious example to take in discussing the ethics of prevention in child health is immunisation. However, this has already been discussed in some detail and I will therefore focus my remarks on screening. Screening procedures have of course expanded greatly in recent years and this raises many questions of rights, benefit, cost advantage, and ethics.

The first question is are we certain that the screening examination concerned will not be harmful to the subjects. Not so long ago, before the Second World War, at least in Belgium, all school children underwent a radioscopic examination each year and thus all screening procedures are not inocuous. This includes examination of IQs because of the importance that parents may attach to the results of this kind of testing which we know to be of very limited and variable significance. A second important question is how serious is the problem we want to screen for? This does not only involve the prevalence of the condition but its duration and level of harmfulness. This may provide a comment about the risk question raised earlier about screening for phenylketonuria – such screening may produce only 10 cases per year in a country like Belgium but the test is cheap and routine and the effects of the biochemical error can be prevented. And this leads directly to the third question – does the medical profession have an answer to the condition being screened for? Is there a treatment or even the possibility of curing this condition or of protecting from the damage it may cause? Fourthly, another important consideration is the scientific validity of the screening procedure. What are the sensitivity and specificity of the tests which can be in a sense contradictory and may lead to different conclusions about appropriate forms of action?

I would like to turn now to mental health issues. Problems of mental health have a high prevalence in children and can reach 12 to 15 per cent of the child population in some countries if we include neurotic manifestations, mental retardation, low IQ, and other conditions such as psychosis. School maladjustment indeed can affect as much as 40 to 50 per cent of all children in certain circumstances. Of course mental health problems are very varied in their appearance and prevalence in society just as society's reaction to them has changed dramatically from one generation to the next. There is a very nice book, written in French under the title of 'L'Art d'Accomoder les Bébés' – loosely translated as the art of educating, cooking, preparing children! In this, the authors review the very contradictory ways in which these problems were tackled. Problems in mental health, even more than those in physical health, are multivariate in character and it is very difficult to establish causal and other related factors.

In this area too, prevention and early intervention may be more efficient than later intervention. If we can cut, for instance, into the mechanism which causes school maladjustment, we are in a strong position to try to prevent the isolation, anti-social behaviour, and eventual delinquency of the children concerned and the adolescents they become. There is a paradox here and a danger in that the earlier we act in prevention, the more difficult it is to identify the children who will benefit most from our action. By intervening early, we lose the ability to define those children who should be taken into preventive action and those who will take care of their problems by themselves. There exists a great variability of psychological conditions and troublesome children, and many may be resolved without any intervention.

There are examples of mental health problems which concern not only the child but also the family. One of these is the very serious and disturbing problem of mistreated battered children which raises at least three difficult ethical issues.

At what level of risk should we provoke a separation of the child, for its own safety? There are cases where this was not done and the child died. On the other hand, most families fear and resent separation, and if we separate the child, it can be very difficult to initiate the serious medical and psychological help needed by the family itself. The dialogue between family and health professional presents another intractable problem – how to prevent recurrence of maltreatment? What is the normal acceptable level of aggressive behaviour? For certain families in some social groups, aggression in the form of physical punishment does not have the same meaning as it might in another family. If we are attempting to help a child and family and we start by giving a normative statement about the harm aggression can do, we risk cutting the channels of communication and jeopardising any possibility of real help. In Brussels, and I think several other cities, another approach is currently being tried. It can be described as primary prevention and its aim is very early diagnosis of high risk mothers during pregnancy. These mothers are then involved in psychological dialogue about their pregnancy and the developing child and we listen to their problems and difficulties and try to assess how help can be provided.

Another interesting issue in this field is the prevention of psychosocial mental retardation, one of the main causes of school failure and probably of later social consequences. Many interesting projects are currently in progress on this subject in various countries. The Heber-Garber project in Milwaukee, USA is very active in helping young families, mothers and children, to cope with educational issues, and to prevent this retardation. This group has succeeded in improving performance so that children previously achieving a development quotient (DQ) of about 80, have attained a level of 100 to 120. This has been done at a very high cost, but it is a project which apparently worked successfully. There is another project in Mons in Belgium, being undertaken by Pourtois and colleagues. Another in Maryland, USA is the PICA project – Programming Interpersonal Curricula for Adolescents – where in a school setting it proved possible to prevent delinquent behaviour. One of the most interesting common denominators of these projects is that they rely to a large extent on self-help, help from neighbours, or help from people in the same social community. The research psychologist or psychiatrist acts as a sort of catalyst and starts off a process which continues without professional input.

One of the most urgent and difficult issues in any ethical consideration of preventive medicine in childhood is how to reach the children of the most underprivileged social groups – the so-called 'fourth world'. There are important projects underway on this in Lorraine, Nancy, Brussels, and elsewhere. Here again there is a very high risk of using a normative approach. It is very difficult indeed to understand the behaviour of people who see things so differently from ourselves and live in such a different way. Values such as time, the keeping of appointments, the organisation of life are viewed in a completely different way. There is a very strong demand for freedom on behalf of this population and this sort of philosophy has been proposed in France by the Quatre Monde movement of Father Brezinski. This has, as a basic principle, the respect of the mental and social freedom of the population. But again this carries a risk which we must confront and evaluate – there were, for example, about 20 destitute people who died from cold last week in Paris. They could have gone for help and care to some social institution, but they chose their freedom and independence. This is perhaps another insoluble ethical dilemma, and it has implications which we should consider for those who work in this particular area. They face some very difficult ethical situations and are constantly confronted with very different value systems which complicate their work and are impossible to resolve without specific training and much discussion.

My final point is to raise the issue of confidentiality in dealings with children and adolescents, predominantly of course the latter. The key question is whether we can or should be sure that we will not tell anybody, in particular the parents, about the difficult things these youngsters have to tell us. This is an immensely complex matter, especially if there appears to be a risk of suicide or of leaving home.

These are just a few of the issues that I hope will encourage discussion of the ethical issues involved in preventive child health.

DISCUSSION

Discussants: Nicholson (Chairman), Canosa, Dunstan, Jeanneret, Knox, Lambiri-Dimaki, Mumuftu, Roy, Strasser, Tognoni, Veatch

Discussion opened with comments on current inequalities and prejudices in health care for children and questions about how we should decide priorities in this field. The two other main issues for discussion were the question of communication and cooperation between disciplines involved in child health and medicine in general, and the need for research in children and the risks and responsibilities entailed.

Evidence is now available on the inequalities between different social groups in terms of physical help and accidents. In Great Britain, Sir Douglas Black produced a report in 1980 which showed that for some sorts of accidents there was a tenfold difference in mortality between social class I and social class V – that is, between the professional families and the manual workers. There are even more glaring inequalities. In South Africa, for example, the infant mortality among black children is at least 10 times higher than among white children.

We also tend to follow societal prejudices and we should perhaps question whether this is ethically the right course of action for us as preventive experts. One example of this is the effect of life expectancy upon our valuation of the life – that is, the child is thought to be more valuable because it has longer to live. If we take an action such as screening for phenylketonuria we count all the years of benefit as well as the discrete benefit of saving a life. And yet, when we move back to the fetus, say an 18 week fetus, this life expectancy effect seems to disappear. The fetus does not carry this valuation. That is a curiously illogical ambivalence or prejudice. It is there in society and we tend to follow it.

The other prejudice, which is perhaps more a medical than a societal one, is that we tend to favour the prevention and treatment of discrete hazards with well-defined mechanisms. We understand the mechanism of phenylketonuria, for example, and it has a discrete taxonomic diagnosis. Yet, there is a great deal we could do relatively simply in pregnancy and the perinatal period to improve the intellectual and physical performance of our children. The use of effective education methods, for example, to reduce smoking in pregnancy and improve dietary intake would increase birthweight and therefore reduce perinatal mortality and the risk of sensory motorneurone defects. In numerical terms the benefit of this type of simple and inexpensive action far exceeds the benefit to be obtained from more costly investment in the prevention of phenylketonuria. Yet the one strategy is so highly valued that it would be unthinkable to withdraw screening for phenylketonuria and the other so undervalued that it is very difficult even to persuade an obstetrician to mention smoking or enquire about smoking habits. Some recent American work suggests that increasing birthweight and similar activities probably contribute only about 20 per cent to the reduction of perinatal mortality that has occurred with improved neonatal care accounting for the other 80 per cent. In Britain the geographical variation in perinatal mortality is almost entirely accounted for by variations in birthweight, whereas the temporal improvement has occurred in all birthweight groups because of an improvement in standard of care. So both factors operate and operate very effectively. In setting priorities for child health, therefore, we must try to consider these issues. In a study in France, reported by Sénécal in 1982, for example, mass screening revealed 80 cases of phenylketonuria and 600 000 cases of maltreated or abandoned children, school absconders, drug addicts, suicide attempts, and so on. Similarly, in 1984 in Spain a programme of mass screening identified 24 cases of phenylketonuria and over 35 000 cases of low birthweight. These imbalances must be a cause for concern.

In this context we must also consider the ethics of teaching and training medical students and where the emphasis should lie in order to prevent some of what we can call the new morbidity or new pathology in developed countries. Measles, mumps, and rubella have practically disappeared from common practice. Yet we are facing new problems of suicide attempts, teenage pregnancy, drug addiction at earlier and earlier stages. There is perhaps a need to sensitise future physicians to social and ethical issues involved in the practice of medicine and to include appropriate topics, such as social philosophy, ethics, sociology, in their curriculum as is already done in a number of countries.

The principle that the child should be among the first to receive protection and care was raised in the context of some very recent philosophical research in the United States on the legitimacy of the role of age in determining health care priorities. There have been several papers published within the last year or two which have examined this question of whether age is legitimate in deciding priorities. Much of the work has been stimulated by a sense that the very elderly get or even deserve to get, low priority because of their age. Assuming that we are motivated by a commitment to provide equality of wellbeing among the population, it makes an enormous difference which of the two following interpretations is given.

Under one interpretation, we want equality of wellbeing at a given moment in time, in which case the infant and the elderly person would seem to get equal priorities. An alternative interpetation has been that we need equality of wellbeing averaged over a lifetime. Since the elderly have had a great deal of wellbeing over much of their life, the direct implication of this argument is that the infant should get high priority. This argument seems increasingly convincing. The goal of a policy, in this case in preventive medicine, ought to be to provide equalities of opportunity of health over a lifetime and the infant who is in jeopardy from the very earliest moment of life, would in this interpretation get special priority in a health prevention programme. This seems to apply directly to the principle quoted by Professor Sand and provides philosophical support for what may seem superficially to be a rather strange notion that the child deserves to be among the first to receive health protection and care.

A further point on priorities is that the chronic mass diseases of middle and old age have been shown to start in childhood and adolescence. Ten per cent of children between the ages of 10 and 14 years already have coronary lesions and the smoking disease may start in teenagers. Evidence of these long-term effects must have immediate relevance for the health of the child in adolescence, and for our decisions on priorities.

One major problem in relation to the ethics of prevention in child health is that of communication of confidences between people of different disciplines, each relating professionally to a family where there is a child at risk. It may be the doctor, the community nurse, the social worker, the probation officer concerned with the family, the school doctor with an older child – each of these individuals may know of the possibility of a child at risk of abuse, but feel bound by a strict interpretation of professional secrecy not to tell. They are never brought together to share their experience until the child has been very badly mutilated or even murdered. This is a problem in Britain at any rate because, I think, of a strict or narrow sense of professional secrecy which needs to be enlarged so that information can be shared among other trusted professions. This question of communication can be enlarged also to include the dialogue between medical and social research findings to try to improve health and social policy. The language of ethics as related to medicine is a language of normative and prescriptive statements. The language of politics is also normative and prescriptive and there is common ground between ethics and politics which could be further exploited to advantage. Changes in the environment to minimise health risks, for example, are largely a matter of political decision. Better communication could help to ensure that these political decisions will be better informed on the ethical and medical principles involved.

On cooperation between disciplines, sociology is a science which could be helpful to investigate ethical issues arising from medical practice and research. Sociology, for example, can help in the diagnosis of socialisation processes by which values about 'health and ill health' are transmitted in the family, at school, and through the mass media with obvious applications in health education. The point was also made that there are differences in practices of referral within and between countries with the emphasis sometimes perhaps on psychiatry, psychology, neuropsychiatry, paediatrics, or sociology. These differences have obvious implications both for health care and outcome and we should be aware of them.

The final issue raised for discussion concerned the need for research to improve the medical treatment of children. In one very small medical school in Canada it was argued very strongly that research should not be carried out in children, even in areas where the risk would be relatively minimal, precisely because the children cannot give consent. The extension of this argument is surely that increasingly effective, non-dangerous medicine is only for consenting adults. Research is of course essential for progress in the field of child health as in any other. And such research is questioned on moral rather than medical grounds. The ethical dilemma here involves the risk attached to the particular research. In assessing the viability of a given research project, the risk is measured against the benefit. In this context there is an important distinction between therapeutic and non-therapeutic research. The former is for the benefit of the patient or subject himself, the latter may provide more benefit for others. We have to minimise the amount of research in children and to allow nothing beyond minimal risk. The United States National Commission for the Protection of Human Subjects of Biomedical and Behavioural Research, defines minimal risk as that which is normally encountered in daily living or in the routine medical or psychological examination of healthy children. Even so defined, minimal is a relative term. On the question of the dangers of using a normative approach to research in child health and the application of results, it was suggested that some attention should be paid to two well-known pathological phenomena, especially related to the fourth world – these are the labelling process and the self-fulfilling prophecy.

CONCLUDING REMARKS

PROFESSOR SAND

The differences in morbidity and mortality between social levels was discussed at length at WHO Europe two weeks ago. It is an important and interesting issue. On the point of deciding priorities between rare diseases and more common conditions, I think that in prevention we must be orientated in both directions. We cannot now stop screening for phenylketonuria, but this should not prevent us from working on low birthweight or other highly prevalent symptoms where preventive action can be taken. I would like also to say a word about our attitudes on the priorities to be given to the minority groups that cannot speak for themselves. In my own case, the paediatric department and geriatric department are next door to one another and we try to work together. It is not a case of either children or the elderly and it is clearly untrue to say the greater the age, the lower the priority. Decisions on priority have to be made but there are many other relevant factors.

The problem of maltreatment of children and secrecy between professional groups is a very difficult one, particularly in countries with a liberal medical tradition with a high regard for personal freedom. In some towns in France and in Belgium – in Liège, for example, and Antwerp and Brussels – teams of health professionals have been set up to try to help in such situations. These are called 'équipes de confiance' and include doctors, nurses, and social workers, working together in a specified geographical area. Many of the preventive activities to which I referred were initiated by doctors or psychologists, but carried out by teachers or volunteers. The Milwaukee project, for instance, was carried out by retired teachers and other volunteers from the region. Many of these projects require commitment rather than qualification and this is an area we could perhaps develop.

ETHICAL ISSUES IN MASS SCREENING PROCEDURES

POVL RIIS

HERLEV UNIVERSITY HOSPITAL, UNIVERSITY OF COPENHAGEN, HERLEV

DR NICHOLSON (CHAIRMAN)

Our next speaker is Professor Povl Riis, Professor of Internal Medicine at the University of Copenhagen, Chairman of the Danish Central Scientific Ethical Committee, and Editor of the Journal of the Danish Medical Association.

PROFESSOR RIIS

In the present context, screening is defined as large-scale diagnostics. Its aim can be primarily orientated towards the individual or towards society and will often be a mixture of the two approaches. The ethics of screening procedures will vary accordingly.

In order to analyse the ethical issues involved, screening can be divided into three groups or categories. The first group concerns screening as a part of large-scale scientific projects aimed at evaluating the effect and value of the diagnostic intervention, or screening applied as large-scale diagnostics without being part of a scientific project. The ethical aspects are similar in principle in these two situations. Informed consent as a fundamental part of the usual doctor-patient or patient/healthy volunteer-scientist relationship, is not accessible in the form of a positive answer from individuals, only at its best as a right to abstain. Furthermore, both the informative and consenting parts of this concept can be weakened in countries and regions with a subtle infrastructure, problems of illiteracy etc, which necessitate the informed consent being given by proxy. Even the demarcation of scientific prevention projects from traditional clinical projects is not always easy, and they share the major ethical concerns, independent of the numbers of patients or subjects involved. In clinical diagnostic trials, for example, prevention is often a part of the scientific approach. And while the numbers involved in large-scale diagnostic trials can be very large, especially in multi-centre projects within and between countries, the numbers involved in centrally administered prevention programmes can sometimes be very small.

The second screening category comprises risk groups, pre-illness groups, and early morbid cases, according to the level chosen. Here the ethics will vary considerably, approaching the ethical demands of clinical practice when one moves from groups with a minor risk to groups of early morbid cases. In this type of screening the presuppositions, information, and consent (at least the right to say no) are crucial too. The preventive or therapeutic consequences of diseases included in the screening programme present possible ethical problems. If no preventive or therapeutic possibilities exist, only prognostic benefits are left. In such cases it has to be considered whether a knowledge of a serious prognosis will not be an intolerable burden to a patient, outweighing the benefits of making it possible for him or her to plan the remaining life in accordance with this prognosis. This emphasises the well-known dilemma in clinical medicine of possessing an answer but not having a question. Moving 'upstream' is often very confusing and can sometimes cause great harm and suffering. The key to personally identifiable data must always be the patient or subject's question or need. Without this key, such information should not be disclosed. On the other hand, screening data can be exploited for epidemiological purposes with little ethical concern. The only exception to this is the possibility of stigmatisation of small diagnostic subgroups even if anonymous data are reported.

The third possible category divides screening not according to course of disease but according to course of life in pre-natal and post-natal screening, with the latter further divided into screening of children and adults. Again, the ethical issues vary considerably from category to category. Special ethical problems can arise in pre-natal screening according to different circumstances. A screening programme may be directed towards all pregnant women – that is, virtually a non-risk group, apart from the small overall risk related to pregnancy in a developed country. It is further influenced by the pregnant woman's possibility of refusing to participate, and by the balance between society's gain through saved costs and the attempts to protect the genetic mass on the one hand, and the autonomy of the individual on the other. The ethical dilemma can be intensified if suspicion arises of reduced support from society to a family who refuse ante-natal screening or abortion in the case of diagnosis of a congenital defect. In the worst case, mass screening might induce a shift in a particular society's attitude towards severe congenital malformations from the idea of Fate to that of a man-controlled, avoidable event, involving an element of guilt. There are examples of such a shift in attitudes and norms stemming from scientific progress – the contraceptive pill and antibiotics leading to a more permissive attitude towards promiscuity, and more recently and in the opposite direction, the new disease entity of AIDS leading to a feeling of alienation among male homosexuals.

The ethical aspects of pre-natal screening will be different if screening is offered only to risk groups – that is, women who are anxious about their unborn child because of earlier malformations among previous children or in family cases. In other words: 'In the beginning was the fear, then comes the method', and not the other way around. Until now, the diagnosis of a risk fetus can, with very few exceptions, only be 'remedied' by abortion. This links pre-natal screening to a destructive intervention quite different from other screening-related interventions. As an important side-effect one has to examine the ethical discrepancy between society's attitude to the large number of abortions carried out in countries with free legal abortion and the selective concern shown on a minority of abortions (approximately 0.25 per cent) resulting from pre-natal diagnosis. Following the different techniques now available – amniotic fluid aspiration, chorion villus biopsy, ultrasonography, chromosome analyses, biochemical assays, DNA probes, and so on – different types of diseases will be looked for and this leads to ethically difficult problems of defining the threshold between abnormal states and conditions acceptable for even minimal levels of quality of life. Information on the sex of the unborn child in cases of non-sex-linked congenital diseases or in healthy fetuses can pose a grave ethical problem, linked as it is to the threat of ante-natal sex discrimination. The introduction of chorion villus biopsy will intensify this problem as the time of diagnosis will move under the time limit of some national laws on free legal abortion.

In summary, we can conclude that ethical aspects of screening procedures and programmes will have to be dealt with according to the same ethical principles already worked out and applied to the patient-doctor relationship and to clinical research.

DISCUSSION

Discussants: Nicholson (Chairman), Blaney, Campbell, Dunstan, Gorovitz, Pinet, Roy, Violaki

Discussion opened with comments on the objectives of screening and the distinction between screening and antenatal diagnosis. The subjects of abortion and fetal therapy were then raised and final comments concerned deficiencies in current medical education particularly relevant to diagnostic and population screening.

Screening is normally taken to mean the application of an economic and simple test to the total population, with the objective of significantly – whatever that means – reducing the size of the particular problem within that population. Screening should not be a situation where use of the service is left entirely to members of the public who could decide to have the particular test whether or not they might benefit. This unfortunately is the situation we have had for many years with regard to cervical cytology. This test is paid for out of public funds but is treated almost as a private service for people who have the time and the application to attend. This usually means it is not the group at risk that is being screened, but the group which is least at risk, the young single female. If a test is going to be applied to a total population in order to reduce significantly a particular health problem, we have to face the ethical problem of how you persuade people to participate.

There is a different ethical emphasis according to whether we talk about pre-natal diagnosis or whether we talk about screening. Screening carries the implication of seeking defects or conditions that can be treated or removed. A case can be made for saying that couples can be offered pre-natal diagnosis of certain conditions in order then to make up their minds whether they wish to proceed with an abortion or whether they wish now to prepare for the birth of a handicapped child. We should, therefore, perhaps avoid the use of the term screening in relation to some of these conditions. Pre-natal diagnosis can be seen as a provision of information and it is perfectly ethical to leave it then to the parents to decide whether or not an abortion is an appropriate decision for them.

It was felt by some that there should be this distinction between pre-natal diagnosis and pre-natal screening. The word diagnosis can be used for an examination of individual patients who presented themselves and the word screening for the systematic application of that examination to a whole population at risk. The clinical consequences of the examination are a matter for decision afterwards whichever process is used, but there should be an objective way of using the two words, diagnosis and screening, which does not depend on subsequent clinical management. However, the term screening is also used for screening in a diagnostic setting, with individual patients. The element which attracts the label of screening is not whether it applies to individuals or populations but that the patient is not complaining about the condition which the examination aims to identify.

Different countries will obviously have different policies for screening and there can be no general rules for procedures and conditions to be sought. However, procedures must be acceptable as valid tests and society has to have some evidence of benefit and about the possibility of false positive and false negative results.

Two possible explanations were offered for the discrepancy mentioned by Professor Riis between society's attitude to the large number of abortions carried out routinely in countries with a liberal abortion policy and the concern shown on the small number of abortions carried out after prenatal diagnosis of some abnormality. The first possible explanation would be that, until the recent tests, such as the chorion villus biopsy test, were developed, abortion for the handicapped was inevitably going to have to be performed relatively late. And there is stronger feeling, for quite obvious reasons, against abortion at the later stage in development than at an earlier stage. A second possible explanation is that the many thousands of early abortions are usually quite anonymous but the handicapped are an identifiable group. Some people may feel the danger of stigmatisation of the group of handicapped who are not aborted, because of this procedure. An example of such stigmatisation was given in the case of screening in Greece for thalassaemia. This has extended to the Greek Cypriot community in North London. Here, if a pregnant woman does not have ante-natal screening for thalassaemia and does not agree to an abortion if she is found to be carrying a fetus with the condition, she and her family are likely to become complete social outcasts from this tightly knit community.

Another ethical problem related to abortion has to be considered. At a recent meeting of the National Ethical Committee in France, chaired by Jean Bernard, the problem of the use of embryos and fetuses for research was discussed. This raises many issues, not least of which is the matter of obtaining consent for such use from a woman or couple in these circumstances. And here we have to be aware that laws are not made for ever and that legislation should vary according to the evolution of society. If ethical issues arise and are in conflict with the existing values of society, society must act accordingly. These are not static concepts and this is perhaps particularly important at a time of such rapid scientific development. It is relevant, for example, to the question of artifical techniques of reproduction. Is there an absolute right, as was stated earlier, to conceive or not to conceive or should we be trying to help those unable to conceive in other ways, such as adoption?

The highly refined ultrasound technique for ante-natal screening has produced a phenomenon of late revelation of fetal defect which can lead to demand for late abortion. In two examples of this from Canada, so-called therapeutic abortions were refused at 30 and 32 weeks on the grounds that the abortion would be of very great danger to the women concerned. This presents a paradox in the use of the term therapeutic abortion when the abortion itself becomes a potential cause of damage to health or even to life.

A recent conference in New York of the Planned Parenthood Association included discussion on how to achieve some clarity on thinking about new possibilities. What do we do, for example, when the abortion fails in the sense that the outcome is a viable fetus, given the capacity of adjacent neo-natal intensive care facilities. What are our obligations and what the permissible behaviour? There is an increasing view that it may be time to stop talking about trimesters and move to a semester system. The distinction is then made between the first half of pregnancy in which the presumption is in favour of a liberal policy toward abortion and the second half of pregnancy in which there is a strong presumption against abortion, unless there are exceptional circumstances.

On Professor Riis's statement that abortion is at the moment the main remedy for a risk fetus, the issue of fetal therapy was raised. This is not yet far developed, although some amazing things have been done, even in terms of surgery. It is, however, likely to make considerable advances over the next 10 years. As it does, we will see an increasing potential conflict between maternal rights to physical integrity and medical duty to treat the fetus as a patient. A foretaste of this can be illustrated by one recent case in the United States, where a woman was ordered by a judge to undergo Caesarian delivery because a normal delivery would possibly have been a danger to her and certainly a danger to the fetus. This could indicate the beginning of a quite different train of thought with acute ethical implications.

The issue of medical education was then raised. The remarks made apply in general to the whole of the content of the workshop but are perhaps particularly relevant to the present topic. In 1984, the President of Harvard University issued a report to the Board of Overseers, the trustees of Harvard University, which contained a scathing indictment of contemporary American medical education. He called for a total transformation in the content of medical education. One of the points that he emphasised was that preventive medicine and preventive health measures have traditionally been virtually ignored in medical education and they should be moved into prominence. He also mentioned the complete statistical illiteracy of medical students and the physicians they become. This is particularly relevant to questions of diagnostic and population screening. The example was given of asking a group of pre-medical and medical students for their interpretation of some hypothetical diagnostic results describing a fairly rare disease. They were provided with information on a test which identifies say 90 per cent of the positives and generates a certain percentage of false positives, given the hypothetical results, and asked to state the likelihood that a particular patient has the disease in question. The mode of response was that the likelihood is about 85 per cent when the actual statistical likelihood is closer to five per cent! Statistics and statistical matters are simply not well understood because they are not taught in any serious way. And we are talking here about a population of professionals whose lives are inextricably bound up with statistical information. So we must all bear in mind the need for constant urging of reform of medical education, in respect both of statistics and of issues in prevention.

CONCLUDING REMARKS

PROFESSOR RIIS

To me screening takes place when we work through the substructure of a health system and reach those who have never considered the possibility of a disease or of carrying a defective child. They have not come to the doctor for a diagnosis of a perceived problem and this is different from the usual clinical situation. It becomes even more difficult when we turn to the quality of a diagnosis made at screening. When we clinicians diagnose a process in the lung, for example, we are likely to say either that it is bronchopneumonia and we can treat it with ampicillin, or it is unfortunately an early tumour and must be operated on. In the clinical situation, where the patient knows or suspects there is a problem, we tend to use this binomial sort of problem orientation. This does not apply in screening because if we identify a problem, it is one of which the subject is not, as far as we know, aware. In this situation – expressed in the language of the lung example – we are more likely to say: 'I can hear something in your lung. We might be lucky, it might be bronchopneumonia, but there is a 15 per cent risk that it could be a cancer and it could be several other things.' Theoretically we should then leave it to the patient or his family to decide on the best course of action. In reality, of course, there is no such value-free information. As clinicians, whether we like it or not, most patients will ultimately ask for our advice on what they should do. This is one of the real practical problems of screening – to know the true linkages between the different diagnoses and the outcome of the analyses. One approach is to do more in risk groups than they ask for, but not give information before we know how to interpret the factors that emerge as side-results.

In Denmark the problem of stigmatisation is exacerbated because some of those participating in the abortion debate are in favour of abortion in those who are not ill and against it in those that might have severe congenital defects. Attitudes to the fetus, to women in society, and to many other societal norms have changed radically within one generation. Our way of thinking in ethical matters and in medicine in general will reflect such changes. Legal abortion is a complicated phenomenon because at the same time we also fight to save babies of 850 grams. So we face two curves, one representing the right to be saved and the other the right not to live because of risk of a congenital disease.

I fully agree that education in preventive medicine and statistics is lacking. As an former teacher of scientific methodology, especially in clinical science, I know well the appalling situation. One can travel around the world as a kind of flying circus, giving courses in medical statistics at a very basic level, and clinicians will view it as a kind of religious awakening to a wonderful new world. Statistics and ethics are seriously linked. An experiment or interpretation of results without knowledge of methodology and statistics is, in itself, unethical.

ETHICAL ASPECTS OF POPULATION CONTROL

HELEEN TERBORGH-DUPUIS

METAMEDICA, RIJKSUNIVERSITEIT LEIDEN, LEIDEN

PROFESSOR VEATCH (CHAIRMAN)

The penultimate paper of this workshop will be presented by Dr Heleen Terborgh-Dupuis from the Faculty of Medicine, Riksuniversiteit, Leiden. Dr Terborgh-Dupuis is an ethicist and lawyer working within the medical setting.

DR TERBORGH-DUPUIS

I have been asked to speak specifically about population control which of course differs in several important respects from preventive medicine. I would like to open with two remarks about the subject. The first is that I do not intend to discuss sexual morality or sexual behaviour as I do not believe either to be relevant in the present context. I take the view that sexual behaviour, having very limited consequences for others, is indeed a totally private affair. This is not the case with family planning, parenthood, and questions of fertility and infertility. The second point is that I do not wish to discuss all the different levels of compulsion by the state. There are many possible methods of coercing or compelling people in a disguised way and it would take too long to cover them and their moral implications satisfactorily.

What I would like to do is to examine the basic moral problem in this field – the problem of the conflict between autonomy and paternalism – and to make some general comments on the conflict between individual rights and the common good, as sought by the state. It may be helpful to distinguish three sorts of individual rights. First of all, there are the classic and well-known rights of freedom – freedom of thought and speech, for example, the freedom of the press, and the right not to be interfered with by the state. Secondly, there are the rights of self-determination, also rights of freedom but much stronger than those in the first category. Thirdly, there are the rights to particular benefits, such as education, health care, and so on. In Holland, these are sometimes referred to as 'positive rights' because they imply active provision by the state. With the first two groups, on the other hand, the government has simply to create a free space for people to act and think as they wish.

The conflict between individual rights and the state's desire to promote the common good, involving if necessary some infringement of freedom rights, has already been discussed in this workshop. But is this the real conflict? Perhaps we should speak rather of a conflict between the individual rights in themselves. Those who wish to claim freedom on the one hand and rights to health care on the other assume the existence of a state willing to provide both that freedom and the health care without limitation. This may not be possible and it may be that those health services can only be effectively provided if people recognise the possibility that the fulfilment of their right to health care might infringe their rights of freedom. Is there not, in other words, an inner conflict within the human rights themselves? The question now becomes one of whether it is morally acceptable for the government or state to limit the so-called freedom rights in the pursuit of health care which implies both an individual and a common good. Is the state ever allowed to know better than the individual? Can the state justify a paternalistic point of view, and if so how? How can we defend an infringement of freedom rights – that is, the right to act as one pleases – in order to promote the right to health care and the common good?

There are, in my view, two conditions which should be met to justify such an infringement. First, there must be a certain level of consensus in society with regard to what is desirable and in the interests of the people. This is difficult but not impossible to achieve. It implies that there are some generally accepted basic human values and carries the danger that we may become locked in an ideological circle. But we do need some basic human values. Let us take the example of two statements: 'Torture is bad for people' and 'Illness is bad for people, health is good for people'. Of course these are value judgments. But could we not also agree on the 'relative' objectivity of the two statements? If so, we may have a possible justification for a paternalistic approach by the state, as long as the second condition is also met. The second condition relates to the consequences of the individual's behaviour. Intervention of the state in preventing or discouraging certain kinds of behaviour can only be justified if that behaviour has undesirable consequences not only for the individual concerned but also for other people or the common good. The essential value of the concept of freedom rights implies that people should be free to act as they like unless they harm others. If they do so and if they also harm themselves, there may be valid justification for an infringement of freedom rights by the state. In many cases, both conditions are met and even seem to reinforce each other. The legal obligation to use safety belts in cars, for example, works not only for the benefit of the individual but also for the common good. The state in this case can know better and is allowed to overrule the individual because it has been demonstrated that the use of safety belts does reduce severe injuries, and if people refuse to use them, the disadvantage is not confined to themselves but applies also to society in general which has to pay the cost.

Another example is in the technique of *in vitro* fertilisation. Before entering moral discussions on this technique, we should first try to prevent the infertility that makes its use necessary. We now know that almost 70 per cent of this type of infertility is caused by previously contracted venereal infections. Should the government do something about that? Once again state intervention can be justified in preventive activities here since such action is in the interests both of the individual and of society.

In conclusion, government actions in the prevention of undesirable individual behaviour can be morally justified. We should not exaggerate freedom rights to the detriment of other human rights such as that to effective health care. And we should speak not only of rights but also of duties. We should assume some sort of reciprocity when we discuss the question of implementation of rights and accept that these carry with them some sort of obligation to society and to the common good.

DISCUSSION

Discussants: Veatch (Chairman), Beauchamp, Campbell, Canosa, Crawshaw, Dunstan, Gorovitz, Karhausen, Knox, Pinet, Roy, Tognoni

Discussion on this paper focussed firstly on the whole question of population control and then moved to general consideration of rights and the concept of the common good.

It was suggested that it might be wise to draw a distinction between a population policy on the one hand, which seems to be assumed in the term population control, and changes in the size or structure of a population which result from individual decisions taken on other grounds. These decisions, for example, concerning contraception and abortion for personal, medical, or social reasons, will affect the size and structure of a population in many ways. But they do not amount to a population policy.

The relationship between the state, society, and ethical judgment in the medical profession can be nicely illustrated by the example of population control. An historical description of the development of population control would allow us to see how medical arguments have interacted with other factors in this particular area. The rationale behind population control is not primarily influenced by either the state or the medical profession. The population solved the problem first, by adopting the methods. In Italy, for example, abortion was adopted in advance of any legislation. The adoption of a particular health policy, therefore, is not always based on moral or medical grounds but results in many cases from general social and economic influences.

Some insight was provided into the current position on family planning and population control in Spain. The birth rate in Spain in the last five years has fallen between 25 and 30 per cent. In some parts of the country the decrease has been as much as 50 per cent. The Spanish Government recently passed a law to make abortion legal under three conditions – rape, congenital malformation or inborn errors of metabolism, and serious risk to the mother's physical or mental health. About two months ago, the head of the department of obstetrics and gynaecology in a very large medical centre was suspended from work because he refused to provide an abortion. There was a great deal of press coverage of the case but it was not reported that the patient involved was a minor and also mentally retarded. Society in Spain is currently facing serious ethical and legal problems in this field. Ninety-eight per cent of the population is Catholic and the Catholic Church forbids abortion and family planning on moral grounds. The Spanish Medical Association recently spoke out against abortion. Yet the state has just legalised abortion on specific social and health grounds. So here we have a complicated mixture of the ethics of the medical profession, personal freedom, and legal and religious aspects which all require to be taken into account. And although Spain has a particularly strict policy on abortion in the European context, it must be noted that an extremely permissive legal attitude to abortion also raises acute and disturbing ethical problems.

The question of arguments based on rights was illustrated by quotations from various declarations on the subject. The first of these comes from the Universal Declaration of Human Rights of the United Nations in 1948: 'No one should be subjected to arbitrary interference with his privacy, family, home or correspondence nor of his honour or reputation. Everyone has the right to the protection of the law against such interference'. However, when it came to the European Declaration of Human Rights, the wording had altered slightly: 'Everyone has the right to respect for his private and family life, his home and his correspondence. There shall be no interference by a public authority with the exercise of this right except such items in accordance with the law and as necessary in a democratic society in the interests of national security, public safety or the economic wellbeing of the country, for the prevention of disorder or crime, for the protection of health or morals, or the protection of the rights and freedom of others'. We can now turn this round and reword it as follows: 'Public authorities in democratic societies may, in accordance with the law and in the interests of all those things, override individual privacy in respect of personal, family life, home and correspondence'.

Thus we started with an absolute statement of right. Then because we had to protect the society that conserves those rights, we had to make some exceptions. In the course of making those exceptions, the right – at least in any absolute sense – disappears entirely. So what do we mean by a right? How can we base any argument on rights when we are then forced to accept that no rights are absolute? Jeremy Bentham stated that talk about rights was nonsense and to talk about natural rights was nonsense upon stilts. But, although much talk about rights is not useful, it does not follow that all talk about rights is nonsense. To say that no rights are absolute and that, therefore there are no rights is to move very far, very fast. The fact that no rights are absolute does not mean that there are no significant respects in which we can make useful reference to the notion of rights. There are rights through law that are clearly defined and well established. We refer to them as legal rights and their meaning is clear. Beyond that, in claiming that a right of a particular kind exists, we do not in general mean that that right is absolute or inalienable. What we mean more typically is that there is a very strong presumption in favour of a particular liberty or mode of behaviour and that strong justification is required to override it. When people can be said to have a right to privacy, for example, we imply not that that privacy can never be invaded, but rather that one who wishes justifiably to invade it, must have strong and valid reasons for doing so.

We must be extremely careful about using the language of rights as the basis of public policy as it can lead to injustice and inequality. An example of this from Canada are claims for Amerindian rights to very large tracts of land that have been in the hands of aboriginal people for many generations.

Rights also carry their practical problems, sometimes very immediate in terms of violence. In Portland, Oregon, for example, 40 per cent of gynaecologists have been drawn into court on various issues, including that of contraception. An amazing and horrifying statistic from the United States is that the sixth most common cause of death among physicians is homicide. This coupled with the fact that 20 US clinics dealing with gynaecological and fertility problems have been blown up on the premise that it was morally 'right' to destroy them, lends an immediacy to our discussion on rights. We should not think that rights are more than they really are. They are never absolute but they can present a strong case, usually based on social consensus, for a certain mode of behaviour.

Use of the term 'the common good' implies some vague understanding of its meaning. But there may be dangers in becoming more specific on this. The existence of a definable item, the common good, if it could be empirically identified by some sort of scientific research would refute any sort of democratic concept of open society. If there is something which we can define as the Common Good, then surely the state should enforce it, whether people want it or not. But can we?

In any case, we should try to articulate a sense of the common good and this may not be as difficult as it may seem if we modify the approach. We can think of ourselves as individuals and members of communities possessing a shared sense of good which is very clear, at least in public health. We can improve aggregate welfare, along with control of disease. While we do not know which particular individuals have benefited from these measures, we do know that we have made advances as a community. That is very different and much more practical and attainable than the idea of a common good identical for each individual, the same for everyone.

CONCLUDING REMARKS

DR TERBORGH-DUPUIS

On the discussion about rights, I can say that for me rights are moral values and are absolutely central to any consideration of ethical issues.

On the dangers of speaking about the identification of the common good and what is good for people, I think that we do this all the time, not only in politics, but also in medicine and many other spheres. We have certain ideas about what is good or bad for people. So why should we be so afraid of making general statements about it? I would challenge any one of you to disagree with the statement that severe suffering is bad for people. What, therefore, is wrong with saying it? If we are going to make progress, we must be prepared to try to define our goals, not as a vague concept but in a more practical and practicable way. The common good may not be so dangerous or so ambiguous as we try to make it.

METHODS AND PROCEDURES OF ETHICAL CONTROL

JEAN F MARTIN

INSTITUTE OF SOCIAL AND PREVENTIVE MEDICINE, UNIVERSITY OF LAUSANNE, LAUSANNE

PROFESSOR VEATCH (CHAIRMAN)

We will now hear the final paper of the workshop from Dr Jean Martin, Deputy Chief Medical Officer of the Public Health and Health Planning Service in Lausanne and Chief of Medicine in the Institute of Social and Preventive Medicine at the University of Lausanne.

DR MARTIN

The issue of control of ethical aspects of health care has been widely discussed in recent years in relation to biomedical research and curative or palliative care. Ethical control of preventive actions has not, however, received much attention, and I would like here to examine some of the relevant questions. As agreed with the organisers of the workshop, I am concentrating on questions raised by the implementation of programmes of preventive action rather than research. Ethical control in practical prevention is a less well-examined area where the answers are more elusive than in research. Preventive research projects tend to be carried out mainly in well-defined conditions in university settings where in the last 15 years ethical control procedures have become progressively routine.

I have tried to look at the issues from the point of view of a public health practitioner, bearing in mind the type of actual situations we now have to confront. In outlining proposals for control, I refer to what appears desirable as well as appropriate and feasible in the current health systems and socio-cultural contexts of developed countries. This is an imperfect world and some of the suggestions may be criticised as being simplistic or unlikely to ensure complete ethical supervision. For this I offer no excuse except to say that I wished to consider practical situations and these are rarely tidy or complete. Similarly, many of the solutions cannot be universally applicable. Although ethics carries with it a sense of concepts which should be valid for all human beings, it is clear that specific control procedures must be adapted to different populations and societies. This being so, I have looked rather for common denominators.

There are several ways in which ethical control in practical preventive medicine differs from that in curative or palliative medicine and most research. First, the relationship, the contract, between recipient and provider of service is not the same in the preventive context. It is usually vague and it is not always clear that the recipient gives a mandate to the provider. Secondly, recipients are usually healthy individuals, at least subjectively. They do not present with a complaint and might therefore be less ready to accept preventive action, even when it aims to promote their wellbeing. Thirdly, the beneficial effects of preventive action often become evident only in the medium or long term. Fourthly, in prevention we are usually dealing with groups of people rather than individuals. This makes it particularly difficult to obtain specific informed consent from all those involved.

In practice, ethical control is not required in the same way and with the same intensity in all cicumstances. In this regard, it is appropriate to consider three main groups of preventive activity. The first is health protection or what we call 'passive' primary prevention. We refer here to measures which, once decided upon in principle, are usually applied by the public authority, without the individual citizen having any influence on them, and, over time, often without the individual even being aware of them. Examples of this kind of prevention include iodiation, fluoridation of the water supply (or, as is the case in Switzerland, of table salt), legislation about water treatment, control of foodstuffs, medical drugs, and other common products, speed limits, obligatory use of restraints in traffic and other such driving regulations, immunisation, and regulations aimed at protecting the environment in terms of land use, building, industrial development, pollution and, so on. The second group of preventive activities includes active primary prevention or health promotion programmes in large groups or whole communities. These are programmes with a large health education component, based in the community and trying to promote behaviour changes and new lifestyles in the population. They are orientated towards problems such as cardiovascular disease, smoking, alcohol abuse, unfavourable nutritional habits, lack of physical exercise. The major ethical question here concerns the prevention/individual freedom interface. To what extent is it acceptable to influence people's actions even when it is for their own good, to what extent can we accept paternalism? The third group of preventive activities is orientated towards individuals and can be described as prevention in personal care. In the practices of physicians or other health professionals, these activities are directed to individual patients or small groups. Some of these relate to health promotion and active primary prevention as described above, although this is not yet particularly common in general practice in many countries. Secondary prevention procedures, such as the Papanicolau smear test, breast examination for tumour, detection of latent or early diabetes or of high blood pressure, are more often performed in this context at present.

Before considering ethical control in practice in these three groups of activities, I would like to say a word about the role of ethical committees. These committees have been created especially in university settings for the principal purpose of supervising research and aspects of curative care. In terms of preventive programmes applied or offered to large numbers of people, ethical committees in practical prevention would not be advising or referring to academic bodies but, in one way or another, to the community. By the same token, they should be representative of the main groups which play a role in the health system in general (see figure). The method of appointing these committees needs care and attention. Normally, the most acceptable – or least unsatisfactory – way is to have such a body designated by government, in consultation with the relevant groups. Another possibility is that a commission chosen by an academic or professional group be entrusted with certain tasks by government, although this might not be as credible a system for the other sectors involved. Such a body, appointed by public authority, would also require a guarantee that it can function independently from government. Ethical control in practice is perhaps simplest in the first prevention group – passive primary prevention or health protection. Here public authority usually takes the measures or proposes them to Parliament, or in some cases, to the people. Several Western countries, for example, have in the past 20 years had popular votes on such issues as fluoridation and obligatory use of restraints in vehicles. It is desirable that authorities at the various levels concerned with health should have or create prevention committees or councils with responsibility for advising on measures to improve health protection of the public. The level concerned is not always the national one, especially in federal

Partners in the health system and in the decisions which need to be taken

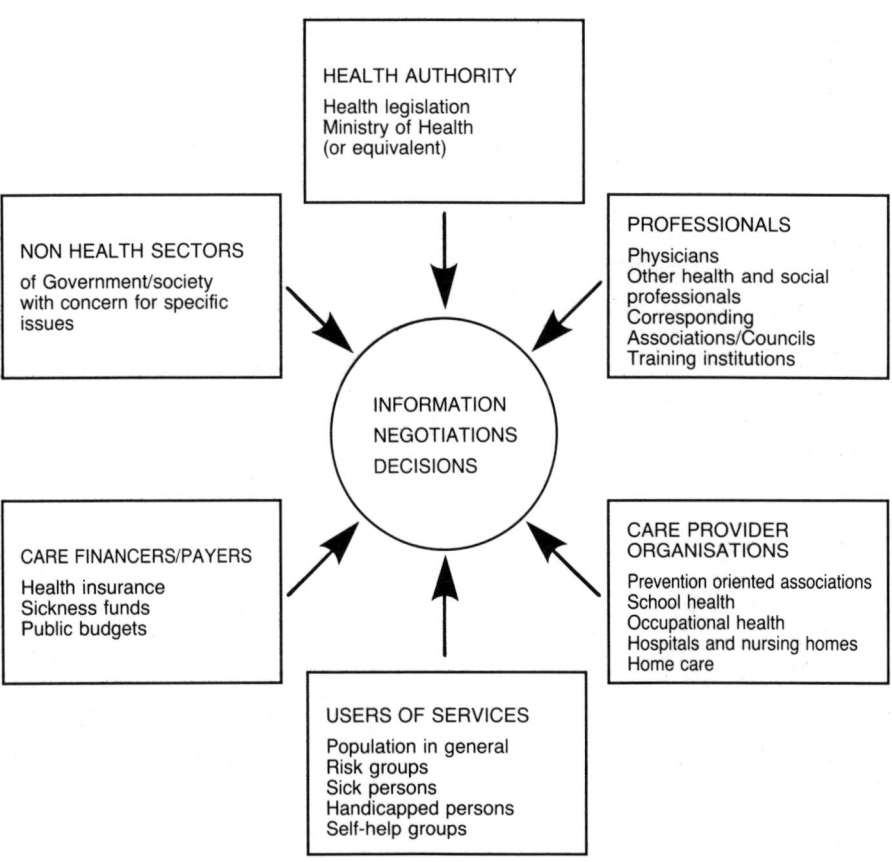

structures, such as the United States (States), West Germany (Länder) and Switzerland (Cantons). These preventive committees should study the technical questions raised by health protective measures. But they should also consider the ethical aspects, possibly through a subcommittee set up for this specific purpose. Government would thus be able to base and justify where necessary its initiatives in this field on competent multidisciplinary advice. The committees would include technical experts, health professionals, ethicists and religious scholars or priests, lawyers, ombudsmen (if they exist), and representatives of the community at large.

Ethical control in community-based active primary preventive activities has to take into account that such programmes are voluntary in essence. People are invited to participate in activities conducive to better health but remain basically free to decline. Successful implementation of such programmes requires the effective participation of many members of the community who must be involved in major decisions concerning it. Such individuals will be members of the local programme committee responsible for running or at least supervising all activities. This committee will also include or work closely with technical experts and will be in a strong position to judge ethical questions that arise. In this type of health promotion activity, one can also count on a measure of informal control by the community itself. No programme can succeed if it runs counter to prevailing attitudes and practices. In our countries, the risks of 'moral terrorism' by advocates of prevention are small indeed. Any attempt to impose new behaviour patterns or lifestyles is likely to meet with indifference or rejection. In a community-based action research project financed by the Swiss National Science Foundation and aimed at preventing cardiovascular disease, for example, it was found in Nyon in the French-speaking part of Switzerland that efforts focussing directly on smoking cessation were not well accepted and very few people registered for such activities. In the same area, a vineyard region where wine is very much part of the social mores, one would not get very far either in an outright attack on wine drinking, and alcohol-related education has to take this factor into account.

Ethical control in individual orientated prevention is governed by the fact that this type of activity takes place mainly in a one-to-one or one-to-few relationship in a doctor's office, clinic, or surgery. It is provided in the same form and within the same setting as curative care and within the same contract between professional and care-requesting individuals. Furthermore, the patient or subject often does not differentiate significantly between personal care with a preventive objective and care for curative purposes. The patient is also free to change care provider if he is dissatisfied with the service received. And although it may be difficult to assess the relevance and quality of care provided, this does represent a protection. Thus the ethical principles that apply in curative or clinical medicine should be observed in this context.

As I have already mentioned, a committee for ethical advice and control appears desirable in the case of passive preventive measures. In practice, it could be entrusted also with supervisory functions for the other areas of prevention. Its advice could then be sought on ethical problems arising in community-based health promotion projects and in personal preventive care. One issue for decision is whether resolutions taken by such a committee should have the value of a decision by the authority. In general, it would seem preferable for the committe to issue recommendations. This would preserve its independence, in maintaining a clear status and mandate – to provide advice on ethical issues. If its resolutions were to be made obligatory, confusion could arise between its role and that of the government.

In summary, ethical control in practical preventive medicine cannot be dealt with in a uniform way. It has to involve the communities it concerns and the representatives of various groups within them. Governments and their administrations are concerned as they implement a number of health protection measures. Ultimately Parliament and the people (possibly through referenda) have to take certain decisions in this regard. There is a need for the creation of committees or councils to supervise the ethical aspects of prevention and to propose new measures when appropriate.

A substantial debate in the community is needed on these issues. For that debate to be useful, however, correct and sufficient information should be available to all sectors concerned – a considerable challenge. Such topics must also be discussed increasingly in the course of the training of concerned professional workers. There are many current health problems which call for a multidisciplinary approach with active communication and collaboration. In the actual training institutions, such as Faculties of Medicine, the necessary changes take place only slowly. Ethical control is one of many themes which demand that an evolution takes place and which could give practical opportunity to illustrate how different disciplines can work together.

DISCUSSION

Discussants: Veatch (Chairman), Beauchamp, Campbell, Canosa, Gorovitz, Knox, Riis, Roy, Tognoni, Zakopoulos

Some unease was expressed about the categorisation of preventive measures into active and passive groups. It is certainly more a continuum than a discrete distinction. There is a range from strong coercion or the construction of barriers through the provision of incentives that may be mild or strong to persuasion or simple advice to adopt a different lifestyle.

The discussion then centred on two closely linked issues – first the question of the committee system and its mode of operation and secondly the relationship between ethics and democracy and the use of referenda. Experience of the committee system in Denmark which has included preventive projects for the past four years has shown that there is a sort of continuum of ethics: the committees appear suitable in the preventive as well as in the curative field. The Danish system has been based on full parity between lay and professional people. Thus they have avoided the single hostage of a woman or a lawyer and have included a very firm and good contingent from the population. Such committees are best organised on a regional basis, covering a geographical area, rather than focussing on a university or hospital. This makes for unified ethical supervision for the whole range of scientific or medical activities available to a geographical population.

It was said also that ethical committees and similar bodies, especially in their application to public health research, work best as advisory rather than decision-making bodies. As soon decisions become mandatory and the element of compulsion is introduced, personal accountability is eroded to a very large extent. And personal accountability is one of the more precise ways of controlling the ethics of research. Another argument for the advisory rather than mandatory mechanism in most cases is the implications for epidemiological research. The example was given of a region with 22 districts, each of which has an ethical committee. If there is a mandatory structure, permission for a research project has to be negotiated successfully with 22 separate bodies. If, on the other hand, the mechanism is advisory, discussions can be held with just one committee who can give approval, subject to possible modifications, for research to proceed. This has the added advantage that responsibility for the ethics and conduct of the project remains with the project leader rather than being taken over by the mandatory bodies.

Some concern was expressed at the notion of resolving ethical conflicts or making ethical decisions by means of a vote. In some contexts this may be exactly the right way to reach a public policy decision about an ethically controversial matter. But there are risks – in some circumstances, for example, slavery has had the support of the majority of the population. And there is also the question of who can vote and who actually votes – it is rumoured that in one Canton in Switzerland, women still do not have the right to vote. In Athens during the time of Pericles, almost 2400 years ago, there was direct democracy. But we have to remind ourselves that only the free people were allowed to vote. If we allow society to decide by means of a referendum what is right and what is wrong, major groups in society may decide in radically different directions. In Canada, for example, an amendment to the criminal law dealing with abortion permitted abortion in cases where the woman's health was in danger, but gave no legal definition of health. It also set a procedural rule that abortions were acceptable also when they were approved by a therapeutic abortion commmittee established in duly accredited hospitals. A practitioner, Dr Morgenthaler, established abortion clinics outside the duly accredited hospitals and was acquitted three times after being brought three times to trial in the province of Quebec. He has just been acquitted a fourth time in the province of Ontario. So ethics by jury is contradicting the ethics of the legislature. Another problem about the referendum method is that there can be a lack of information or of a full awareness of the issue from the population as a whole. In Great Britain, for example, it is clear that if there were a referendum, there would be a return to the death penalty for capital crimes. A majority of members of parliament in both main parties, who are much better informed about the implications of returning to the death penalty, are opposed to it and vote against it. This is a good example of the importance of representative democracy – important decisions are taken by elected representatives who themselves must gain the information to make well-informed decisions.

The opposite opinion in favour of the use of the referendum was also expressed. In Italy, the death penalty was actually removed as the result of a referendum. And there may be a place for linking this kind of popular vote on certain issues with the use of representative committees. There is certainly a need for flexibility to decide the best system in a particular context and for clear and open-minded thinking about the issues involved in practical prevention. The notion of participative democracy is implicit if not explicit in Dr Martin's paper – the idea that democracy works better when we can increase the participation of all citizens in the decision-making process. The Oregon experiment, described earlier in the workshop, is a clear example of this, although outside the state structure. There is much to be explored in the notion of a democracy in which an increasing number of people are able to participate in an informed manner, on decisions which affect themselves.

It is important that we recognise the tension introduced by democratic procedures in public health. There seems to be a sentiment that democracy and ethics are somehow pitted against one another, that one is a bad method and one is a good method. This may be because we have long experience of democracy and we see its disadvantages as well as its benefits. With ethics, on the other hand, we always deal with a sort of ideal world. This is not a practical or productive way of looking at ethics or politics. Since ethicists are not legislators, we do not know how good a job they might do in comparison with our democratic representatives.

There is and must be a distance between ethics and politics. We must leave ethics free, in some sense, to seek improvement in the character of political decision-making. Public health, on the other hand, particularly in its practical application, needs a much livelier sense of democratic possibilities because this is where our ethics are put into practice and theory becomes reality.

CONCLUDING REMARKS

DR MARTIN

I persist in believing that there are significant differences in ethical control between curative and preventive medicine, particularly if we talk of active prevention programmes. These include many non-medical activities, aiming at the promotion of health through behaviour changes. Prevention includes also arrangements of the social, technical, or physical environment in which we live. It is not possible to regulate this type of activity in the same way as clinical research.

I have tried to deal with the ethics of prevention being implemented – that is, the action societies or groups might take as routine measures to improve or promote health. It would have been much simpler to deal with research in preventive medicine where the terms, settings, and limits are relatively clear and defined. The former is a different problem and one that is much less studied and much less tidy.

I agree that the active-passive prevention categorisation is a simplification and the reality is much more of a continuum. However, my intention was to provoke discussion. I also wanted to underline the fact that once the decision has been taken by whatever means to accept a so-called 'passive' measure – be it compulsory immunisation, seat belt legislation, pollution control – then the individual citizen has little influence on subsequent events and is therefore in a passive situation. Ultra-passive measures are of course often counter-productive – prohibition of alcohol in the United States, for example, did not work.

I agree that ethical committees or similar bodies should in most circumstances be advisory rather than mandatory.

I have no good response to give on the fact that one Canton in Switzerland (60 000 people out of six and a half million) still denies voting rights to women. There have been moves to try to impose from outside a change in the constitution of this particular canton by a federal mechanism, but this was rejected by our national parliament in order not to infringe the freedom of the smaller community.

The referendum or popular vote cannot be a universal solution to our difficult decisions. But I still believe that we must sometimes resort to that kind of mechanism, in spite of the fact that it brings problems as illustrated by the abortion example from Canada. We must certainly strive for flexibility and interaction and this is one of my main points. Much of what we have been discussing is how to find the happy medium, the 'juste milieu'. In practical prevention there are no universal rules, there is no such thing as a group that routinely knows best.

CLOSING REMARKS

ROGER BLANEY

It is a very great privilege to have the last word in this workshop on ethical issues in preventive medicine. I happen to have this honour because I am a member of the Planning Committee on this project and of the Panel for Epidemiology in the EEC which has helped to support this workshop.

There are 17 different countries represented here, and I hope that the way we have worked together and pooled our ideas on these very difficult issues will result in an interesting and valuable published report of the proceedings. We also have representatives of a wide range of specialties and skills - physicians, epidemiologists, sociologists, specialists in public health, ethicists, theologians, economists, lawyers, journalists, experts on health policy.

I know we all have been very impressed with the amount of hard work achieved. The workshop over the past two days has run from early in the morning until late in the evening, and I am not going to detain you very much longer. We have dealt here with a wide range of interesting and important issues. We have discussed the theory of ethics and the theory of public health, the recurring question of human rights, the issue of duty, the gap between ethical judgment and ethical behaviour. We have been reminded of the distinction between preventive medicine and individual medical care, and of the differences of prevention in research and prevention in practice. We have looked at the transfer of benefits, confidentiality, the right to privacy, informed consent, and the relevant but so far nameless concept which I shall call blaming the victim – that is, making the person who has incurred harm to health through his or her own behaviour take the financial consequences. It is a tribute to all participants that these issues have been discussed in such a civilised and productive way from often very different points of view and attitudes. If when you return home, you should care to put a short summary of the proceedings into a relevant journal or publication, it would be most useful in spreading ideas and promoting discussion of this important subject.

My final and very pleasurable task is to thank you all together and individually for giving up your valuable time to contribute your particular skills and expertise to the workshop. I would like also to thank each of the chairmen who have handled these proceedings so tactfully, efficiently, and productively. Finally, I come to our Greek hosts, and first of course to Dr Doxiadis to whom we are so very much indebted for making this workshop possible and for the superb organisation and excellent hospitality we have received in Athens. He has been most ably assisted in this by Mrs Catherine Zahopolou who has done a tremendous amount of work in the background. On your behalf I would like to thank them most sincerely and to include in this the other Greek participants who have contributed so much to the discussion and made us so very welcome in their country. The recording team have also done an excellent and unobtrusive job which is crucial to the quality of the final report. In summary I would like to thank everybody who has contributed to making this workshop the success it has undoubtedly been.

SPYROS DOXIADIS

Very briefly, on behalf of my country and of the Foundation for Research in Childhood, I would like to add my thanks to all of you, and especially to the members of the Planning Committee, for all the work you have done and the honour you have paid us in coming to Athens and contributing in various ways to this very valuable project.

INDEX

A

Abortion	2, 9, 15, 60, 85, 85, 87, 88, 89, 92, 100, 101
Acropolis	13
Aesculapius	6
AIDS	85
Alcoholism	20, 22, 34, 38, 63, 96
Ampicillin	88
Antibiotics	85
Aristotle	7, 13, 17, 62
Asbestosis	77
Aspirin	57
Atherogenesis	55
Atherosclerosis	55
Aversion methods	60, 61, 62, 63

B

Bacteriuria	28, 29
Baedeker's Advice to Travellers (1894)	65, 66
Bentham, Jeremy	26, 27, 28, 93
Bezafibrate	55
Bhopal	34
Biliary atresia	69
Bioethics	9, 36, 41
Bismarck	27
Board of Overseers (Havard University)	88
Brain death	67
Breast cancer	23, 76
Bronchopneumonia	88

C

Cancer	22, 23, 48, 61, 64, 68, 73, 75, 76
Cardiovascular disease	49
Censorship	67, 68
Cervical cancer	22
Chadwick, Edwin	20, 26, 28
Cholera	20, 21
Christian medical ethics	15, 17
Cigarette smoking	37, 39, 40, 41, 42, 43, 49, 56, 60, 61, 64, 76, 77, 81, 82, 96
CIOMS	15, 41, 57
Clofibrate	54, 55, 58
Club of Rome	41
Cognitive abuse	60, 61, 62
Commission of the European Communities	3, 4, 5
Common good	91, 93, 94
Community physician	2
Company physician	74, 75
Confidentiality	20, 21, 22, 47, 48, 49, 50, 51, 74, 75, 80, 102
Congenital hypothyroidism	23

Congenital Rubella Syndrome 48, 51, 52
Contraceptive pill 85
Coronary heart disease 54, 55
Council of Europe 5

D

Declaration of Hawaii 1977 13
Declaration of Helsinki 1964 12
Declaration of Sydney 1968 13
Deontological ethics 6
Directorate of Health and Safety in Luxembourg 5
Drug addiction 22, 57, 81

E

Economics of prevention 42–45
E E C Working Party 47, 48, 49, 68
Embryo 13, 87
Emphysema 60
Environmental issues in health 4, 23, 34, 55
Ethical issues .. 2, 3, 5, 7, 8, 9, 10, 12, 13, 14, 15, 17, 20, 22, 23, 25, 29, 34, 44, 47, 50, 51, 52,
        54, 58, 60, 68, 70, 71, 72, 73, 74, 75, 76, 78, 79, 80, 82, 85, 87, 92, 93, 95, 98,
        100, 101, 102
  Ethical Review Committee 1
  Ethics Committee (French 1983) 5
  Ethics of consequence or utility 6, 7, 8
  Ethics of duty 6, 7, 8
Evolution 14
European Community 3
European Parliament 4
Euthanasia 2

F

Fenofibrate 55
Fluoridation 48, 61, 96
Foundation for Research in Childhood 3, 4, 103
Freud, Sigmund 7

G

Genetic effects 73
Gout 26
Graunt, John 26
Guillain – Barré Syndrome 67

H

Haemophiliacs 22
Health care 4, 12, 43, 60, 81, 82, 83
Health education 38, 59–64, 66, 67
Health promotion 4, 59–64
Heber-Garber Project USA 80, 83
Hippocratic approach to disease 6, 11
Hippocratic tradition 9, 15, 17, 47
Hume, David 5, 8
Hygeia 7

I

Institute of Child Health 1
International Commission on Radiological Protection 77
Ischaemic heart disease 55

K

Kant, Immanuel 6, 7, 8
Kidney stones 26
Kuhn 14

L

Lakatos 14
Lung cancer 64

M

Malarial fever 65
Measles 26, 48, 68, 81
Media 65, 66, 67, 68, 69, 70, 71
Mental health 78, 79, 80, 81
Mentally defective newborn 2
Metaphysic of Morals 7
Mexico 34
Montesquieu 41
M R F I T trial 55, 56
Mumps 81
Musgrave 15
Mutation 11, 13, 14, 15, 17

N

National Ethical Committee (France) 87
National Health Service (Britain) 12
N A T O 3, 68
N A T O Science Council 4
Neural tube defects 52
Nichomachean ethics 7
Nuremberg Code 12

O

Obesity 60
Occupational health 72, 75
Oregon Health Decisions Project 36, 37, 38, 40, 69, 100

P

Panel for Epidemiology in EEC 102
Paternalism 14, 21, 34, 38, 49, 62, 90, 91, 96
Pericles 100
PICA Project (USA) 80
Phenylketonuria 76, 79, 81, 83
Placebo 54, 55
Planned Parenthood Association 87
Plato 8
Pollution control 34, 96, 101
Population control, ethical aspects 90–94
Preventive medicine   2, 3, 15, 19, 20, 21, 22, 23, 25, 26, 27, 28, 29, 32, 33, 42, 43, 47, 54, 56, 68, 71, 75, 76, 78, 80, 82, 84, 88, 89, 90, 95, 96, 98, 101, 102
Public health 7, 25, 28, 29, 30, 32, 33, 34, 36, 77, 93, 100, 102
Public health legislation 32–35

R

Radiation 34, 44, 72, 73, 76, 77
Research 12, 46, 47, 49, 50, 51, 52, 55, 57, 78, 85, 87, 93, 95, 99, 101
Resource allocation 12
Revolution 15, 17
Rights 3, 12, 13, 14, 16, 18, 40, 41, 51, 92, 93
Rosen, George 27
Rubella 23, 48, 51, 52, 81

S

Science Council of NATO 3
Sclerosing panencephalitis 68
Screening 21, 29, 75, 78, 79, 84, 85, 86, 87, 88
Scurvy 27
Seat belts 29, 30, 34, 39, 52, 91, 101
Sensory motorneurone defects 81
Seveso 34
Sexually transmitted diseases 33
Smallpox 23, 33
Smith, Adam 27, 28
Snow, John 20
Southwood Smith, Thomas 26
Stott, Nigel 63
Sulphur dioxide 75
Supreme Court of the United States (1905) 10
Surrogate motherhood 5, 19, 34
Swine Influenza 67
Swiss National Science Foundation 98

T

Thalassaemia 87
Therapeutic medicine 2, 3
Transfer of benefit 21, 22
Transplants 40
Treatise on Human Nature (1739) 5
Tuberculosis 33
Typhus 26

U

U S National Commission for the Protection of Human Subjects
of Biomedical and Behavioural Research 83
US National Institutes of Health 1
Utilitarian ethics 6

V

Vaccination 9, 10, 23, 33, 39, 43, 48, 50, 51, 52, 66, 67, 71, 78
Vitamin A 57, 58

W

Warnock, Dame Mary 5
Warnock Report 5, 12, 29
Whooping cough 23, 66, 57
World Health Organisation 3, 4, 23, 32, 33, 35, 39, 41, 57, 63, 83
World Medical Association 12, 13